A DEVELOPING DISCIPLINE

Selected Works of Margaret Newman

D1714454

A DEVELOPING DISCIPLINE
Selected Works of Margaret Newman

Margaret A. Newman
PhD, RN, FAAN

Professor, School of Nursing
University of Minnesota
Minneapolis, Minnesota

NATIONAL LEAGUE FOR NURSING PRESS • NEW YORK
Pub. No. 14-2671

Copyright © 1995 by Margaret A. Newman
Published by
National League for Nursing Press
350 Hudson Street, New York, NY 10014

Printed in the United States of America.

ISBN 0-88737-638-X

Library of Congress Cataloging-in-Publication Data

Newman, Margaret A.
    A Developing Discipline : selected works of Margaret Newman /
Margaret A. Newman.
            p.   cm.
    Includes bibliographical references and index.
    ISBN 0-88737-638-X
    1. Nursing—Philosophy.   2. Health—Philosophy.   I. Title.
    [DNLM: 1. Nursing—collected works.   WY 16 N554i 1995]
RT84.5.N4793   1995
610.73′01—dc20
DNLM/DLC
for Library of Congress   94-23657
                                                                      CIP
This book was set in Bembo by Publications Development Company.
The editor and designer was Nancy Jeffries. The printer was Northeastern Press.

Cover design by Lauren Stevens.

To
MARTHA
who made the difference

Contributors

Sharon Autio, M.S., R.N.
Mental Health Specialist
Minnesota Department of Human Services
Minneapolis, Minnesota

Sheila Corcoran-Perry, Ph.D., R.N., F.A.A.N.
Professor
School of Nursing
University of Minnesota
Minneapolis, Minnesota

Gerri Lamb, Ph.D., R.N., F.A.A.N.
Director, Community Nursing Organization
Carondelet Health Care
Tucson, Arizona

Frank Lamendola, M.S., R.N., C.S.
Doctoral Student
School of Nursing
University of Minnesota
Minneapolis, Minnesota

Cathy Michaels, Ph.D., R.N.
Associate Director, Community Services
Carondelet Health Care
Tucson, Arizona

Susan Moch, Ph.D., R.N.
Associate Professor
School of Nursing
University of Wisconsin—Eau Claire
Eau Claire, Wisconsin

A. Marilyn Sime, Ph.D., R.N.
Professor
School of Nursing
University of Minnesota
Minneapolis, Minnesota

Contents

.

Prologue

With a great deal of pleasure I have pulled together some of my writings reflecting the development of the discipline. I must admit I have enjoyed reliving the exciting times these steps represent. In 1971, when I wrote "Nursing's Theoretical Evolution," I shared it with a psychologist colleague who was a history of science buff, and he was clearly envious of nursing scientists as we embarked on this journey—he saw us as being on the brink of important discoveries.

Since books are printed and (usually) read in a linear fashion, I have tried to organize my work in some orderly sequence. But each time I thought I had captured the logical order, something would pop up out of order. The first would be last, and vice versa. I finally realized that the content was like the waves of an ocean, reaching a peak and cascading forward only to fall to the water below, surge backwards and arise again and again. So I ask the reader to keep that in mind in the continuing themes that arise repeatedly. From a broad perspective, it is clear that there is an overall progression toward articulation of the theory, research, and practice of our discipline. The successive parts of the book each represent the seamless whole of TheoryResearchPractice but with varying emphasis at different points in time.

I ask the reader's tolerance of my early sexist language. To add [sic] every place I used "man" to mean human or the then "impersonal" pronoun in the masculine form would, I think, disrupt the flow of ideas. You will note that I (as well as others) learned along the way that man does not mean woman. In other instances, the vision of the emerging paradigm was hampered by lapses into old paradigm language. I have tried to alert the reader to the latter limitation.

In 1977, I was asked by the editor of a university alumni magazine to write an article on the status and future of the nursing profession. Considering this an opportunity to speak to a wide audience of readers, I worked diligently to identify and substantiate the factors I thought to be of major significance to our developing discipline: moving from subordinance to medicine to authority in nursing practice, establishing academic doctoral programs as the highest degree in the field, and beginning to clarify the focus of nursing science. With much apology, however, the editor rejected the manuscript on the basis of a reviewer's comments that the ideas set forth, particularly as they related to a new concept of health, were "dangerous" if taken seriously. I surmised that this reviewer came from the perspective of the medical paradigm. And while the editor also had asked for input from nursing colleagues, there still was not sufficient support to warrant her publishing the article. I was disheartened and filed it away for another day. That day has come. As I look back over my published works, I think they reflect the developing practice, education, and science that I referred to in 1977. As a prologue to these collected works, I want to share some excerpts from the 1977 manuscript.

First, the movement from subordinance to medicine to authority in nursing practice:

"The dependent subordinate role, which to many is the image of nursing, is better understood within the context of the role of women in general. Women in nursing were caught in what Adams (1971) has called the compassion trap, the idea that woman's primary social function is to provide tenderness and compassion. In the past, educated women tended to cluster in the helping professions and become involved in housekeeping tasks on behalf of society. There was the insidious notion that the needs of others should be women's major, if not exclusive, concern, and along with this the idea that there was some sort of virtue in subordinating individual needs to the welfare of others. Women have been restrained from taking action on their own behalf for fear of negative repercussions on others that they were protecting. . . . Ashley's (1976) historical study of nursing illustrated the ways in which hospital authorities (primarily men) played upon the dedication of nurses (primarily women) and convinced them that it was their *responsibility to the patient* to work long hours for low pay, and so on. One reason for acceptance of this kind of responsibility, according to Adams, is women's need to fit into the system and to get involved, and therefore, willingness on the part of women to use the characteristics that they have developed—such as tenderness and nurturance—in subordinate roles.

"But nurses have become increasingly dissatisfied with this subordinate role and have recognized the futility of trying to serve three masters—the hospital administrator, the physician, and the patient—probably in that order. . . . Another factor in the conflict is the fact that the hospital is an illness-oriented care facility, whereas nursing is becoming increasingly health-oriented. Practice solely within the hospital setting . . . is focused primarily on a limited phase of the total process, and many nurses choose to have a more ongoing relationship with the client."

Nurses were beginning to establish authoritative roles for themselves by developing private and group practices. Kinlein, perhaps the best known nurse to hang out her shingle at that time, described her reasons (as quoted in the 1977 paper):

I knew I would have to explain the frustration I had experienced as a professional nurse before setting up the practice; my search for the key to the problem; and the ultimate exit from the labyrinth of activities subsumed into the aggregate known—wrongly, I believe—as "medical care." In that maze I could never identify a movement from "here" to "there" that I could call nursing. The "here" and "there" were always set by someone else, and I was always practicing between the two points.

. . . the episodic nature of illness in the health continuum, contrasted with the ongoing nature of health, plays havoc with the traditional concept of being under a doctor's care after a limited period of contact with the doctor—a situation resembling the somewhat unavailing circumstance of being cared for by remote control. Care by a physician is needed intermittently, sporadically, throughout life. The physician gets to look at the individual's health continuum mainly on those isolated occasions when symptoms of illness appear. In keeping with the concept of self-care practices, care by a nurse is needed on a more continuing basis. The nurse views the health continuum of an individual in its entirety, and when and if illness occurs, she views that illness in the context of the individual's total health picture as she, through her nursing care, has learned to know it. Thus nursing, because of its quality of continuity, which is the essence of nursing care—assumes an umbrella-like form that encompasses the other health professions. (Kinlein, 1977)

Group practices were being formed by nurses, prominent among which were nurse-midwifery practices that focused on assistance with preparation for childbirth and labor and delivery for normal, healthy women.

Another major step forward in the development of the discipline, as cited in the 1977 manuscript, was in the area of education:

"Recognizing that an essential factor in being able to offer high quality, health-oriented care was through knowledge, nursing leaders have worked diligently since the turn of the century to move nursing into the mainstream of higher education. Their efforts have not been without opposition. Ashley's study revealed that physicians wanted conscientious, bright nurses *without* an education, or knowledge of their own, so that they would have no basis for questioning their dependence, subordination. Hospital administrators, too, wanted to maintain control of nursing education, since the supply of nursing students was often used in lieu of graduate nurses and, therefore, yielded profit for the hospital (Ashley, 1976). Nurses, too, then as today, opposed this movement toward independence through education.

"Even though progress has been slow, the educational standards accepted by the profession today encourage programs within institutions of higher education at all levels: associate degree for the practice of nursing technology, baccalaureate degree for professional practice, master's degree for advanced practice,[1] and doctoral degree for teaching and research. Whereas in 1970 there were only five doctoral programs in the United States, at the present time [1977] there are approximately sixteen such programs,[2] with a number of others in various stages of development."

And with the development of doctoral education in nursing came the burgeoning of knowledge specific to nursing:

"The development of nursing theory has reflected the pattern of growth of the profession, i.e., a movement from dependence on other disciplines to identification of knowledge specific to nursing. . . . In 1970, Rogers set forth a conceptual framework as a foundation for the development of nursing science. Other nursing theorists offered variations of a common theme: a holistic examination of person-environment relations throughout the life span, with nursing's purpose being to facilitate this process. Crucial to Rogers' conceptual model is the idea that health and illness are not separate entities and, therefore, are not to be studied separately, but are reflections of the changing patterns of the life process. . . .

"Viewing health and illness as fluctuations in patterns of energy exchange precludes our looking at them separately. The conditions that have been regarded as health and illness can be seen as constantly changing patterns: some of which are harmonious, some of which are discordant, some of which are organized, some of which are disorganized, but all of which necessitate being considered as an ongoing exchange. The peaks and troughs of this pattern might be considered the times when the pattern and organization of an individual become increasingly [inefficient][3] until the situation is regarded as illness. It is possible that even in this situation the 'illness' can provide the tension,

---

[1] My position on professional education, then and now, is described in Chapter 20.
[2] Currently there are 61 academic doctoral programs in nursing.
[3] Substitute "disorganized."

or shock, which redirects the energy pattern of the individual and thus brings about a more harmonious, free-flowing pattern. Consider the function of, say, a high fever, or an emotional crisis, or the accident which occurs at a particularly crucial time. These, and many other critical incidents, may produce the shock that facilitates the individual's movement from a pattern that was ineffective for him into another pattern better suited to his needs.

"Understanding of the pattern and the process is needed in order to know when and what intervention is indicated. Diagnosis based solely on pathology of systems and parts obscures the total pattern. Attention to individual parts and alteration of the parts serve to keep us forever missing the forest for the trees. It maintains the activity of changing the original pattern without knowing what we are changing, like being caught in a maze, choosing one turn or the other without knowing where we are going. Total perspective is needed in order to visualize the pattern and make knowledgeable choices.

"It is this kind of understanding of the dynamic pattern of the life process that is the objective of nursing science. We seek to utilize a holistic approach in the discovery and elaboration of patterns . . ."

We have come a long way since that paper was written. Throughout our history we have been plagued with mixed paradigms. Nightingale sought to clarify the difference between the perspective of Medicine and that of Nursing. In Part One of this book, we take a step back into our recent history to clarify the perspective of the nursing paradigm and pinpoint the current focus of the discipline. Part Two addresses the dilemma encountered when methods derived from the old paradigm were used to try to examine the holistic, dynamic phenomena of the emerging paradigm. The integrality of pattern to the paradigm introduced by Rogers was acknowledged long before Rogerian scientists identified and used a methodology of pattern to describe the unitary, transformative paradigm of nursing science and practice.

The new paradigm of health being addressed from all sides of the academic and professional world is nowhere more apparent than in nursing. My odyssey in the development of a new concept of health is traced in Part Three. The experience of research aimed at identifying pattern brought me to the realization of the praxis nature of nursing science.

We have been slow to resolve professional issues of education and practice that have existed throughout our modern history. In Part Four, I include my thoughts on some of these lingering issues that have arisen again and again. Perhaps the gathering storm of health care reform will catapult the nursing profession into a position of first-order service as we enter the 21st century.

REFERENCES

Adams, M. (1971). The compassion trap—women only. *Psychology Today,* November, 71–103.

Ashley, J. A. (1976). *Hospitals, paternalism, and the role of the nurse.* New York: Teachers College Press.

Kinlein, M. L. (1977). The self-care concept. *American Journal of Nursing, 77,* 598–601.

Rogers, M. E. (1970). *An introduction to the theoretical basis of nursing.* Philadelphia: F. A. Davis.

Note to Reader

Although we have standardized the format in this volume, certain differences in writing style reflect the time and context in which each article appeared.

PART ONE

The Emerging Structure of the Discipline

M y interest in tracing the development of nursing as a professional discipline began with the realization that we needed to
differentiate the foundational knowledge of our discipline from that
of the other disciplines closely related to nursing. In spite of
Nightingale's clear direction for the development of nursing science,
we wandered about for three-quarters of a century in search of
research questions specific to nursing. During this period, world
wars and economic depression kept us preoccupied with recovery
and stabilization. During the past two decades, however, we have
emerged as leaders in a pro-active conceptualization and study of
health and caring.

The development of science is not an orderly affair. The product
looks orderly but the process often moves in multiple directions,
reversing itself, repeatedly, as the focus is narrowed and becomes
clearer. The papers in this section reflect this search for a definition
of the discipline—for both the substance and the syntax.

Only recently have we understood the paradigm of health as heralded by Nightingale. In our alignment with the medical model and
related health sciences, we accepted the concept of health in a negative sense—the *absence* of disease. Even though there was an intuitive
sense of health as the *whole,* we failed to recognize the importance
of the interactive, unitary nature of the nursing phenomenon. Then
Martha Rogers' conceptualization of unitary human beings as the
essence of nursing turned us back to the path set by Nightingale.
Since then, we have proceeded to develop a science that is truly
nursing.

Questions about the nature of nursing science prompted an analysis of the prevailing paradigms and focus of the discipline. That step takes us a long way toward clarifying the parameters of the discipline.

CHAPTER ONE

Nursing's Theoretical Evolution

Margaret A. Newman

THE NEED FOR knowledge which is specific to nursing has been recognized since the beginning of modern nursing. Florence Nightingale wrote:

> I believe . . . that the very elements of nursing are all but unknown . . . are as little understood for the well as for the sick. The same laws of health or of nursing, for they are in reality the same, obtain among the well as among the sick. (Nightingale, 1859, p. 6)

The elements which Nightingale identified and attempted to explicate focused on the environment, nourishment, and observation of the patient and on the interpersonal relationship between the nurse and the patient. Even then, participants in nursing confused knowledge of pathology with knowledge of the laws of health. In her attempt to clear up the confusion, Nightingale explained:

> Pathology teaches the harm that disease has done. But it teaches nothing more. We know nothing of the principle of health, the positive of which pathology is the negative. . . .

Reprinted with permission from *Nursing Outlook,* 20:449–453, 1972. Based on a paper presented at the Fifth Annual Clinical Sessions, New York University Division of Nursing, December, 1971.

It is often thought that medicine is the curative process. It is no such thing; medicine is the surgery of functions, as surgery proper is that of limbs and organs. Neither can do anything but remove obstructions. . . . Surgery removes the bullet out of the limb, which is an obstruction to cure, but nature heals the wound. So it is with medicine; the function of an organ becomes obstructed; medicine, so far as we know, assists nature to remove the obstruction, but does nothing more. And what nursing has to do, in either case, is to put the patient in the best condition for nature to act upon him. (p. 74)

Although over a hundred years ago our charge was clear, the direction we have taken in search for nursing knowledge has led us at times away from our responsibility. Only within the past decade have we begun to discover the kinds of information that will assist us in establishing optimal health for man, in sickness and in health.

HISTORICAL DEVELOPMENT

Throughout most of the past century, the approach to nursing was based largely on medical knowledge. Nurses, taught by physicians, were instructed in what physicians thought they needed to know to carry out the medical regimen for the patient. Even the advent of university education for nurses did not change the approach, for curriculums were organized by medical specialty areas. To some extent, this organizational focus persists today.

Another approach to nursing knowledge has been pursuit of the educational process and method. The earliest opportunities for nurses to pursue graduate education were provided by schools of education. The nursing leaders who were prepared in this way thought that the key to improving the quality of nursing care was in improving nursing education (McManus, 1961). Consequently, the research these nurses pursued related primarily to educational and, to some extent, administrative problems in nursing.

Along with the increase in the number of collegiate programs in the early fifties came a growing awareness on the part of nursing faculty of the need for scientifically based knowledge specific to the nursing process. A major step in directing the attention of nurses to research was accomplished with the publication of the first issue of *Nursing Research* in 1952. One of the purposes of this journal, as stated in the first issue, has been to stimulate research in nursing.

An overview of the categories of research and concerns reported in *Nursing Research* during the past 20 years suggests the trends of nursing's theoretical evolution. (Frequencies reported are based on the major articles of the journal and the first-named author.) The magazine's expansion from an original three-times-a-year publication to its bi-monthly status has been accompanied by change both in the quantity of research published and in its content and quality. For example, during the early period, the number of studies that emphasized the role and characteristics of nurses comprised approximately 32 percent of the articles. At the same time, studies relating to the nursing process and the behavior of man accounted for only about 12 percent. Since 1968, although the number of studies emphasizing the functions and characteristics of nurses continued at approximately 24 percent, the number relating to nursing process and the behavior of man has risen to approximately 36 percent.

The change in types of contributors to *Nursing Research* through the years is also indicative of the changes that have taken place in theory development. Whereas 36 percent of the contributors in the 1952–58 period were non-nurses and 26 percent were nurses with doctorates, only 16 percent of the contributors since 1968 have been non-nurses and the proportion of articles contributed by nurses with doctorates has risen to 49 percent.

The large proportion of non-nurse contributors during the early period may explain the bulk of studies on functions and characteristics of nurses. During those years nurses tended to turn to social scientists for help in studying nursing. This approach resulted in restatement of nursing problems as social science questions, with nurses studying nurses, rather than nursing. Wald and Leonard point out that the "pure" scientist was trained to pursue his own discipline and "it might have been expected that he would help nurses develop his discipline rather than nursing practice" (Wald & Leonard, 1964).

APPROACHES TO NURSING THEORY

Concern about nursing theory, which began to become evident in the early sixties, has received considerable attention since 1968. During this period, three main approaches to the discovery of nursing theory emerged: (1) the "borrowing" of theory from other disciplines with an intent to integrate it into a science of nursing; (2) an analysis of nursing practice situations in search of the theoretical underpinnings; and (3) the creation of a conceptual system from which theories could be derived.

Theory from other disciplines—Since 1962, when the federal government started funding the nurse-scientist program to enable nurses to study in other disciplines for the purpose of relating their theory to nursing, the number of nurses who have received doctorates has increased considerably. In exercising the diligence necessary to attain competence in these other disciplines, however, nurses who pursued this type of research preparation have been confronted with a problem in maintaining an intimate relationship with nursing. Although many theories from other disciplines are relevant to nursing, the testing of these theories within the framework of another discipline relates the data more clearly to that discipline than to nursing.

Dorothy Johnson has said that knowledge from the basic sciences is relevant to nursing but that the knowledge needed for nursing practice is incomplete until "we learn to ask . . . nursing questions about events in nature of specific concern to us" (Johnson, 1968). One of the purposes of encouraging nurses to obtain research preparation in related disciplines was to provide a means for enlarging the research potential of nursing faculties. Since this purpose has been accomplished to some extent, supporters of this approach to the development of nursing theory are now beginning to recommend the development of doctoral programs in nursing, with the accompanying emphasis on research of nursing questions (U.S. Health Manpower Education Bureau, 1971).

Practice theory—The second approach, that of analyzing nursing practice in search of conceptual relationships, has gained support since 1968. Wald and Leonard exhorted nurses to direct their attention toward building knowledge directly from a systematic study of nursing experience. They asserted that nursing is a professional practice rather than an academic discipline and that the purpose of a practitioner-scientist is to study ways to achieve changes—changes in patients' responses to such experience as hospitalization or other health measures. They believed that theory of this type could best be derived from and tested in the actual nursing arena (Wald & Leonard, 1964).

One of the problems inherent in an analysis of the nursing situation is the lack of agreement on answers to such questions as: What is nursing? What is the specialized role of the nurse? Only three years ago, at a conference organized for the purpose of synthesizing a theory of nursing, the participants, who were considered leaders in theory development, found these questions stumbling blocks to the advancement of theory basic to nursing (Norris, 1969).

Most recently, in a critique of current nursing theory, Walker begins her discussion with what she considers "the leading question in a science of nursing, that is, What is occurring in nursing?" (Walker, 1971). After a century of asking ourselves that question, we are still not much closer to our goal of nursing theory.

A conceptual system—Much of the confusion about what we should be studying was eliminated, in my opinion, when Rogers identified the phenomenon which is the center of nursing's purpose: MAN (Rogers, 1964). It sounds simple, yet many a graduate student will attest to the difficulty of reorganizing one's thinking about man in order to consider him a unified being and not as a composite of organs and systems and various psychosocial components. The clear-cut delineation of man as the focus of nursing gave direction for the development of theory that is not just relevant to nursing, but basic to nursing.

Thus, a conceptual framework of nursing theory was born. Confident in her designation of man as the phenomenon which is the focus of nursing's purpose, Rogers reviewed the available literature in an effort to identify basic assumptions regarding man and determined that the following statements could be accepted as true:

- Man is a unified whole possessing his own integrity and manifesting characteristics more than and different from the sum of his parts (wholeness) (Rogers, 1970, pp. 46–47).

- Man and environment are continuously exchanging matter and energy with one another (open system) (p. 54).

- The life process evolves irreversibly and unidirectionally along the space-time continuum (unidirectionality) (p. 59).

- Pattern and organization identify man and reflect his innovative wholeness (pattern and organization) (p. 65).

- Man is characterized by the capacity for abstraction and imagery, language and thought, sensation and emotion (sentience) (p. 73).

On the basis of these assumptions, she proceeded to synthesize a conceptual model of man and from there to formulate some general principles from which theories of man can be derived and tested. The relationship of Rogers' conceptual system to data is shown in Figure 1.1.

Hempel, in emphasizing the importance of developing a system of concepts from which general explanatory and predictive principles can be formulated, points out that "science is ultimately intended to

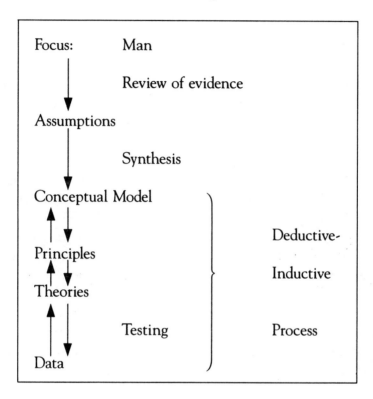

Figure 1.1 Relationship of Conceptual Model to Theory and Research.

systematize the data of our experience. . . ." (Hempel, 1952, p. 21). He perceives a scientific theory as similar to a complex spatial network: the concepts represented by the knots and the unifying principles represented by the strings. Using this network, the scientist can proceed back and forth in the system to observable data and thereby expand the explanatory power of the system (Hempel, 1952, p. 36).

Other theorists in nursing have called for a conceptual system from which nursing theory can be derived (Batey, 1971; Brown, 1964). King has recently proposed four ideas as the conceptual base of the dimensions of nursing: social systems, health, perception, and interpersonal relations. She agrees that the basic abstraction of nursing is the phenomenon of man and his world. The selection of her conceptual base is rooted in her belief that "nurses, in the performance of their roles and responsibilities, assist individuals and groups in society to attain, maintain, and restore health." More specifically, "man functions in *social systems* through *interpersonal relationships* in terms of his *perceptions* which influence his life and *health* (King, 1971). Although on the surface King's system may appear to be quite different from that proposed by Rogers, comparison of statements from the two positions reveals a certain amount of congruity (see Table 1.1).

The principles and postulates identified by Rogers and the premises formulated by King indicate that there is some agreement in the evolving theoretical framework from which hypotheses are being derived and tested and the data therefrom are fed back into the system. The comparisons are by no means complete, either for these two theorists or for other nursing theorists whose formulations may provide additional elaboration of the system. The examples are selected to illustrate

Table 1.1 Comparison of excerpts from Rogers' *An introduction to the Theoretical Basis of Nursing* and King's *Toward a Theory of Nursing*

Rogers	King
The principle of reciprocy: The human field and the environmental field are continuously interacting with one another. The relationship . . . is one of constant mutual interaction and mutual change (pp. 96–97). Basic assumption: Man and environment are continuously exchanging matter and energy with one another (p. 54).	The dynamic life process of man involves a constant restructuring of the real world. The transactions. . . that occur in human interactions are an exchange of energy and information within the persons involved (intrapersonal) and between the individual and the environment (interpersonal) (pp. 87–88).

Table 1.1 *Continued*

Rogers	King
The principle of synchrony: Change in the human field depends only upon the state of the human field and the simultaneous state of the environmental field at any given point in space-time (p. 98).	. . . thus action results from factors in the situation and in the individual at any point in time (p. 88).
Man is a unified whole possessing his own integrity and manifesting characteristics that are more than and different from the sum of his parts (p. 47). The human field possesses it own identifiable wholeness. . . it maintains identity in its everchanging but omnipresent patterning (pp. 90–91).	Man as a composite of mind and body reacts as a total organism to his experiences which are viewed as a flow of events in time (p. 88).
Helicy: . . . the life process evolves unidirectionally in sequential stages . . . is a funciton of continuous innovative change growing out of the mutual interaction of man and environment along a spiraling longitudinal axis bound in space-time (pp. 99–101).	Time is an irreversible process in the life cycle . . . (p. 88).
Man is characterized by the capacity for abstraction and imagery, language and thought, sensation and emotion (p. 73).	Man is a social being. Through language man has found a symbolic way of communicating his thoughts, actions customs, and beliefs over time (p. 88).

that a conceptual system of nursing focused on man is evolving similarly in the minds of nursing theorists and does provide meaningful direction for research. As Rogers has said, "The science of nursing aims to provide a body of abstract knowledge growing out of scientific research and logical analysis and capable of being translated into nursing practice" (Rogers, 1970, p. 86).

The fruitfulness of this conceptual approach to theory development is borne out by the research which has been conceived from ideas based on the wholeness of man's constant interaction with his environment. A series of studies of the effect of the stimulation of total body movement on man have resulted in an evolving theory of movement or motion (Earle, 1969; Neal, 1968; Porter, 1971). Other studies are beginning to outline characteristics of man's spatial and temporal awareness and have implications for his continuous reciprocal interactions with his environment (Felton, 1970; Newman, 1972; Rodgers, 1971; Schlachter, 1971).

Continued exploration of patterns of stimulation are introducing evidence regarding man's capacity for maintaining his pattern in an ever-changing environment. Again, those examples are only a few of the rapidly growing number of studies designed to test the theory of man, with the ultimate purpose of identifying laws regulating this continuous interaction of man and his environment. Knowledge of such laws would then guide nursing practitioners in their goal which is, in essence, to help man achieve his maximum health potential.

THEORY OF THEORIES

Proponents of practice theory assert that theory for a profession must go beyond merely describing, explaining, and predicting a particular phenomenon. Dickoff and James have described four levels of theory: (1) factor-isolating theory (classification); (2) factor-relating theories (situation-depicting); (3) situation-relating theories (predictive); and

(4) situation-producing theories (prescriptive) (Dickoff & James, 1968). Theory, they assert, must provide conceptualization intended to guide the shaping of reality to a profession's purpose. Situation-producing theory, they believe, incorporates the other three levels of theory and, in addition, prescribes the desired outcome of a situation and the activities necessary to produce that outcome. Inherent in this approach is the assumption that the "desired" outcome can be identified.

Nursing is referred to, from time to time, as a learned profession, an applied science, and a practice discipline—somehow with the connotation that these terms have different meanings. Each of the terms, however, has two components: one which indicates the rigors of scientific inquiry, and another which implies a commitment to service. The development of theory for nursing, therefore, is likely to proceed at more than one level of generalization. At present, nursing theorists are working primarily at the descriptive and predictive levels, but the possibility of a prescriptive level exists.

There now appears to be consensus among nursing theorists that nursing is concerned with assisting man to maintain optimal health throughout his life process. There is also some agreement regarding the conceptual framework of nursing. Whether the theory evolves inductively from ideas conceived in clinical practice or deductively from broad generalizations within the theoretical framework does not seem particularly important. What *is* important is that the nursing investigator determine the relationship of her study question to the overall conceptual system in nursing and thus expand and elaborate the system by the testing of theories that have derived from it.

VALIDATION OF THEORY

One of the problems we face in nursing is the need for more valid methods of measuring the variables of our research if we are to learn anything about the reality of the world in which we live. The rigidly controlled experimental studies necessary for baseline studies do not adequately explain the totality of man's interaction with his environment. Field work studies, on the other hand, may be of equally questionable validity. If the phenomenon of man's interaction with his environment is to be described, explained, and predicted in such a way that it is applicable to man in his environment, we must continue to seek new methods of measurement.

ON THE THRESHOLD

Nursing is coming of age. We have established a viable conceptual system—one that provides us with clear, relevant guidelines for theory-building and research. We are no longer overly concerned with ourselves as nurses. Concerned with the phenomenon of man, we are beginning to understand man. We no longer are completely dependent on other disciplines for the knowledge of our practice, but neither are we completely independent. We are beginning to realize our own potential for discovering a particular kind of knowledge that is relevant to other disciplines and essential to nursing. The problem of the past has been the dearth of nursing knowledge. The problem of the future will be the acceleration of that knowledge.

REFERENCES

Batey, M. V. (1971). Conceptualizing the research process. *Nursing Research, 20,* 296–301.

Brown, M. I. (1964). Research in the development of nursing theory. *Nursing Research, 13,* 109–112.

Dickoff, J., & James, P. (1968). Theory of theories; a position paper. *Nursing Research, 17,* 197–203.

Earle, A. (1969). *The effect of supplementary postnatal kinesthetic stimulation on the developmental behavior of the normal female newborn.* Unpublished doctoral dissertation. New York University.

Felton, G. (1970). Effect of time cycle change on blood pressure and temperature in young women. *Nursing Research, 19,* 48–58.

Hempel, C. G. (1952). *Fundamentals of concept formation in empirical science.* Chicago: University of Chicago Press.

Johnson, D. E. (1968). Symposium on theory development in nursing; theory in nursing; borrowed and unique. *Nursing Research, 17,* 206–209.

King, I. M. (1971). *Toward a theory of nursing* (pp. 21–22). New York: Wiley.

McManus, R. L. (1961). Nursing research—its evolution. *American Journal of Nursing, 61,* 76–79.

Neal, M. V. (1968). Vestibular stimulation and the developmental behavior of the small premature infant. *Nursing Research Report, 3–1,* 3–5.

Newman, M. A. (1972). Time estimation in relation to gait tempo. *Perceptual and Motor Skills, 34,* 354–366.

Nightingale, F. (1859). *Notes on nursing: What it is, and what it is not.* London: Harrison and Sons.

Norris, C. M. (Ed.). (1969). Nursing theory conference, 1st proceedings. Kansas Medical Center, Department of Nursing Education.

Porter, L. S. (1971). Physical-physiological activity and infants growth and development. In *American Nurses' Association seventh nursing research conference, Atlanta, Mar. 10–12.* New York: American Nurses' Association. Unpublished doctoral dissertation. New York University.

Rodgers, J. A. (1971). *The relationship between sociability and personal space preference among college students in the morning and in the afternoon.* Unpublished doctoral dissertation. New York University.

Rogers, M. E. (1964). *Reveille in nursing.* Philadelphia: F. A. Davis Co.

Rogers, M. E. (1970). *An introduction to the theoretical basis of nursing.* Philadelphia: F. A. Davis Co.

Schlachter, L. (1971). *The relation between anxiety, perceived body and personal space and actual body space among young female adults.* Unpublished doctoral dissertation. New York University.

U.S. Health Manpower Education Bureau. (1971). *Future directions of doctoral education for nurses.* Report of conference held in Bethesda, MD, Jan. 20, 1971. Washington, DC: U.S. Government Printing Office.

Wald, F. S., & Leonard, R. C. (1964). Towards development of practice theory. *Nursing Research, 13,* 309–313.

Walker, L. O. (1971). Toward a clearer understanding of the concept of nursing theory. *Nursing Research, 20,* 428–435.

CHAPTER TWO

The Continuing Revolution: A History of Nursing Science

Margaret A. Newman

THE DEVELOPMENT OF a science, contrary to what one might assume, is not a smooth, orderly process. The beginnings center around a vague discontent regarding phenomena for which there are no available explanations. Moreover, the identity and nature of the phenomena themselves are not very clear. Nevertheless, there is the conviction that there is something there which needs to be identified, described, and explained, and persons concerned with the same phenomena begin to examine them in some sort of systematic manner.

The process of the development of a science for a profession has some inherent advantages and disadvantages. One of the advantages is the great body of experiential data which provide a wealth of tacit knowledge (Polanyi, 1962) regarding the phenomena of inquiry. One of the disadvantages is the tendency of practitioners to view this phenomenon in a limited way, thereby decreasing the possibility of gaining new insights. It is this latter ability, the ability to view phenomena from different perspectives, that marks progress in the development of a science or, as Kuhn (1970) phrases it, revolutions in scientific thinking.

Reprinted with permission from *The Nursing Profession: A Time to Speak* (pp. 385–393), edited by N. L. Chaska. Copyright by Mosby-Year Book, Inc., St. Louis, MO. Originally published by McGraw-Hill, 1983.

Nursing has had its share of revolutions in the way in which the scientific base of practice is viewed. Nightingale's explication of the phenomena of nursing's concern perhaps marks the beginning of the systematic inquiry and the identification of these phenomena. The purpose of this paper is to trace the major emphases of nursing's thinkers from Nightingale to the present and to illustrate how the shifts in thinking mark progress in the development of nursing science.

Before looking specifically at nursing science, however, I would like to begin by examining the development of science in general.

A preliminary definition of science could be "the process of knowing." There are, however, many ways of knowing: by faith, by authority, by experience—or by systematic, controlled investigation, which some call the scientific method. Most would agree that science is not developed by faith, authority, or experience alone, but even the scientific method, which is more acceptable in scientific circles as a way of knowing, is fallible. We find, to a large extent, what we are looking for; we are limited by the ability to see; and we are limited by the inability to think beyond the prevailing perspective of the day. For these reasons, Popper (1965) would add to this definition of science that the process of knowing is developed by the processes of challenging and questioning. Popper says one can have confidence only in those theories that cannot be overthrown or rejected, and, therefore, the most important contribution that one can make to a theory is to try to refute it, to devise the most stringent test possible, so that if the theory stands up under that kind of testing, greater confidence in its validity may be assumed (1965, 3–65, 215–250). Further, Kuhn, in his analysis of the great discoveries throughout the history of science, sets them as points of radical shifts in the way of viewing things:

> . . . a new theory . . . is seldom or never just an increment to what is already known. Its assimilation requires the reconstruction of prior theory and the re-evaluation of prior fact, an intrinsically revolutionary process that is seldom completed by a single man [sic] and never overnight. (1970, 7)

The preliminary definition of science then may be expanded: it is a process of knowing, a process of challenging, and a continuing revolution. A familiar example serves to show how this process works. There was a time when people thought the world was flat. (Considering how long the world has been around that was not very long ago—approximately 500 years; most of what we know about the world has been developed in that short period of time.) The theory that the world is flat was based on very limited observations. But as the science of mathematics began to be developed, or redeveloped, someone came along and speculated that the world was round. Columbus and his associates checked the theory out and found that it is so, and after a while, it became common knowledge that the planet we live on is a finite sphere. But even so, people of that day were convinced, primarily because of their religion (knowing by faith), that they were the center of the world and that everything revolved around them. Therefore, the world had to be the center of the universe, with the sun and other planets revolving around this planet—again, a limited view of things. Then Copernicus came along and projected the theory that the sun is the center of this universe and that this and all the other planets revolve around the sun. This is a good example of a paradigm shift.[1] Copernicus was looking at the same sun and planets but seeing them differently. Of course, nobody listened to him for a long time, but eventually, on the basis of the calculations of other astronomers, this new view of relationships was accepted. Toward the end of the seventeenth century, Newton put forth this theory of force, or the law of gravity, which was thought to be the ultimate in explaining the laws of the physical world. With the advent of better telescopes, however, people found that some of the predictions of

---

[1] According to Pelletier: "Paradigms impose order upon basically random phenomena. A paradigm is a model of reality, and it gives rise to a philosophical predisposition that directs and interprets the scientific activitiy of its adherents. Its implicit judgments about the nature of reality include some and exclude other phenomena from scientific inquiry" (1978, 37).

Newton's theory were not true. Then in the early twentieth century, Einstein was able to explain things that Newton's theory could not explain. At this point, Newton's theory became a special case in a broader, more comprehensive theory.

A new theory disposes of the mistakes of the old theory. In order to devise a new theory, the scientist must be able to perceive that something is amiss, that something does not quite fit, and then, rather than explain it away within the limits of the old theory, be prepared to look at things in an entirely new way.

In science in general and in nursing in particular, the question keeps coming up: "Are we moving toward one big theory?" In view of the way science has progressed thus far, the answer appears to be "no." One theory contradicts and, in some instances, replaces the other. Einstein's theory contradicts Newton's. Newton's had previously contradicted Galileo's. Agassi describes it this way:

> . . . Galileo's theory said that gravity is the same everywhere. Newton said that this is not quite true; gravity decreases the farther away you go from the earth. In Newton's theory, gravity acts at a distance. Einstein said that this is not quite true; the force of gravity moves outward from a body with the speed of light.
>
> We can say that Galileo's theory or Kepler's theory is a good approximation to Newton's theory, and Newton's theory is a good approximation to Einstein's theory. That is to say, the results we get from Newton's theory are nearly the same as the results we get from Einstein's theory under normal conditions. And Galileo's theory gives results which are nearly the same as the results we get from Newton's theory under normal conditions. But for astronauts, Newton's theory holds good while Galileo's does not. And with high-speed rockets, Newton's theory does not hold good at all, while Einstein's theory is fine. (1968, 147)

The old theories are approximations of the new ones and, as illustrated, are still useful in certain situations. The new theories go beyond the old theories and explain things the old theories could not explain. The process is one of evolution and accretion rather than accumulation.

So, too, the process has evolved in the shifting of theories throughout the history of nursing. A theory can be thought of as "one, powerful idea" (Popper, 1965, 58). From this standpoint, the progress of science can be viewed as a history of ideas: therefore the purpose here is to highlight the predominant ideas, or theories, which have influenced nursing since the time of Florence Nightingale.

The domain of nursing has always included the nurse, the patient, the situation in which they find themselves, and, the purpose of their being together, or the health of the patient. In more formalized terms, or in the jargon of the day, the phenomena of our concern—the major components of the nursing paradigm—are *nursing* (as an action), *client* (human being), *environment* (of the client and of the nurse-client), and *health*. The *nurse* interacts with the *client* and the *environment* for the purpose of facilitating the *health* of the client. It is within the context of these four major components and their interrelationships that theory development in nursing has proceeded. (See Figure 2.1.) Theoretical differences relate to the emphasis placed on one or more of the components and to the way in which their relationships are viewed.

The first major emphasis in the development of nursing science, based on Nightingale's work, was given to *environment*. Nightingale (1859) viewed disease as a reparative process, the effort of nature to remedy a process "of poisoning or of decay," and she viewed the suffering which accompanied disease as being the result of deficiencies in the environment (1946, 5). In her own words, nursing "ought to

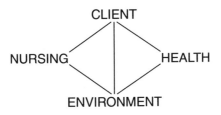

Figure 2.1   The Nursing Paradigm.

signify the proper use of fresh air, light, warmth, cleanliness, quiet, and the proper selection and administration of diet . . ." (1946, 6). The objective of these activities was the health of the patient. Nightingale's approach might be diagramed as in Figure 2.2.

Nightingale equated the science of health with the science of nursing, and based on the most pressing problems confronting her in the Crimea, she focused her efforts on the development of knowledge of the environmental factors she considered essential to health. She also included three other categories of nursing knowledge: observation of the patient, personal hygiene of the patient, and communication skills; but her major emphasis by far was that of controlling the environment.

This emphasis on environmental factors continued well into the twentieth century. Nursing practice was associated with the care of the ill. Medical science had little to offer in terms of curative treatment. The knowledge of nursing practice, therefore, emphasized altering the environment to render it conducive to healing. As important as this factor is, it was not sufficient.

The next impetus to the development of nursing science does not appear to emerge until the middle of this century. Recognizing that I have done only a superficial review of the nursing literature of the first half of this century. I do not find much activity during that period aimed at the advancement and testing of new ideas. It is reasonable to

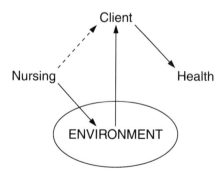

Figure 2.2   Schematic of Nightingale's Approach to Nursing.

assume that nursing leaders were preoccupied with improving nursing education and were convinced that, by so doing, the way would
be cleared for the advancement of nursing science. At the same time,
the demands of two world wars took priority in terms of accelerated
education and practice within acute care centers, with little time for
the scholarly activities of contemplation and analysis.

At the end of this period, however, in 1948, Esther Lucille Brown's
report on nursing education was published, and first among her recommendations was the "need for nurses to study and analyze nursing
functions" (Dolan, 1973, 277). Shortly thereafter, in 1952, the first
research journal in nursing, *Nursing Research,* was published, and the
die was cast for establishing a scientific basis for nursing practice. Even
so, the research efforts of the next decade revealed a great deal of uncertainty as to what to study and analyze, and, as a matter of fact,
Brown's recommendation may have contributed to the confusion.
Many fledgling researchers took her literally and focused their studies on the more obvious functions of nursing, i.e., the techniques employed by nurses in the performance of their responsibilities. After a
decade or so of this type of research, it became clear that the accumulation of such studies was not contributing in a noticeable way to
the understanding of nursing practice.

An era of concerted effort toward the development of nursing science emerged in the fifties and early sixties. The emphasis shifted
from environmental factors to the nature and purpose of the *nurse-
client relationship* (see Figure 2.3). Recognizing that nursing was concerned not merely with doing things for patients in relation to their
discomfort or disability, but also, and perhaps primarily, with the nature of the ongoing interpersonal processes, a number of nursing theorists began to identify these processes more specifically. Peplau (1952)
brought the interpersonal theories from psychiatry into the realm of
nursing and provided a basis for nurses to begin to analyze the process of their interaction with patients in terms of its therapeutic quality. Similarly, Orlando (1961) utilized communications theory in
describing what she termed "a deliberate nursing approach." Later,

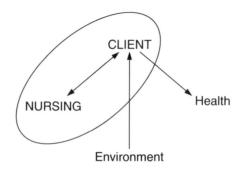

Figure 2.3   Schematic of Emphasis during the 1950s and Early 1960s.

but in the same context, King (1971) began to explicate the complex transactional process occurring between nurse and patient.

Other theorists during this period emphasized the purpose of the nurse-client relationship. In seeking licensure for professional nursing, the profession became preoccupied with defining nursing and trying to differentiate the nature of nursing practice from that of medical practice. Henderson's (1966) definition of nursing is perhaps the most frequently noted—doing for the patient what he cannot do for himself with the intent of promoting independence. Similarly, Orem (1971) conceptualized nursing as the promotion of self-care in the patient. Johnson (1961) identified equilibrium, or dynamic stability, as the goal of nursing care. Roy's (1970) adaptation theory states that nursing's role is that of facilitating the adaptive potential of the patient.

All of these theorists have concentrated on situations in which clients are incapacitated in some way and require the assistance of someone else to supplement their own resources until they can again be independent, maintain self-care, establish equilibrium, or adapt to the situation. Most of these theorists view health and illness on a continuum, with the purpose of nursing being to move the client toward health. Here the emphasis is clearly on the *client,* the person adjusting to changes in himself or herself or in the environment (Figure 2.4).

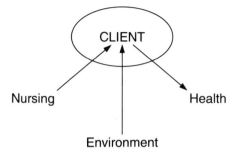

Figure 2.4   Schematic Showing Shift of Emphasis to Client.

Rogers' (1970) conceptualization provides another shift and emphasizes the unitary nature of man and the inseparability of man-environment. She sees the purpose of nursing as the promotion of symphonic interaction between man and environment and views health and illness as simply expressions of the life process. This view differs considerably from that which is based on man's adaptation to the environment. In Rogers' view, both man and environment are exerting their influences simultaneously, and the process is one of mutual evolutionary change. Even so, the emphasis in Rogers' framework (Figure 2.5) is on an understanding of man, the client, within his or her environment. This she sees as the focus of nursing's concern.

Currently there is increasing emphasis on the concept of *health* (Beckstrand, 1978; Newman, 1979; Smith, 1979). Health has been seen as an essential component of all nursing frameworks from the time of Nightingale to the present (Figure 2.6). Each of the earlier explications of health has moved us a little closer to the views set forth today. Nightingale equated health with nursing and admitted that it was an unknown entity. We have moved from a conceptualization of health that depicts it as absence of disease to increasingly dynamic concepts: health and illness as a continuum (Roy, 1970), health and illness as expressions of the life process (Rogers, 1970), health as a process of human growth and development (King, 1971), health as

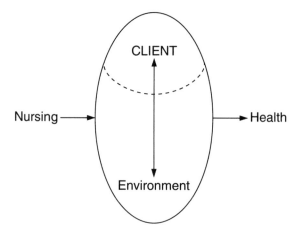

Figure 2.5   Schematic of Rogers' Emphasis.

the expansion of consciousness (Newman, 1979). Much work is needed in the elaboration and exploration of factors in the client–environment relationship which relate to health. Beyond that, theory must be developed to direct nursing action toward facilitating the process of health.

As the earlier discussion of the development of the science of physics demonstrated, we see that what each theory contributed was

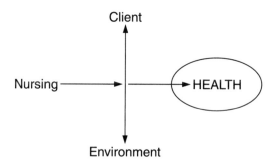

Figure 2.6   Schematic of Current Emphasis.

an approximation of the next theory. No one theory said it all. One theorist picked up where another left off. Each new theory came about when someone saw that something was missing in the old theory. As we look at the various emphases in nursing theory through the years, we can begin to see that what the theorist chose to examine reflected the needs of that particular time, whether it was the lack of proper sanitation and the lack of medical treatment for infectious disease in the late nineteenth century or the increasing numbers of people surviving traumatic injuries and developing chronic, debilitating diseases in the mid-twentieth century. The emphasis on controlling environment shifted to an emphasis on rehabilitation, which in turn gave way to an emphasis on prevention and finally to an emphasis on facilitation of health. Some theorists looked primarily at the nurse-client interpersonal process, others concentrated on understanding the complex processes of the human being as a unit, and others extended that thinking to include interaction with the environment. Finally, health, an integral component of all these interactions, is being examined as a dynamic process fluctuating across the life span.

As already pointed out, some of the theories contradict each other. This however, does not negate the usefulness of the various approaches in certain situations. It does mean that one has to determine under what conditions the theory applies. I would suggest that one of the factors determining the applicability of a theory is the temporal frame of reference. For example, if one is viewing a relatively short time frame, the adaptation model might apply, whereas in a longer time frame, phenomena would be apparent that could not be explained by adaptation alone.

In the early stages of the elaboration of various conceptual models in nursing, there was a tendency to view the models set forth by theorists as competitive or to place relative values on them. This situation is consistent with Hardy's assertion that nursing is in the preparadigm stage of scientific development, a stage "characterized by divergent schools of thought which, although addressing the same range of phenomena,

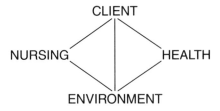

Figure 2.7 Schematic Predicting Emphasis in the Future.

usually describe and interpret these phenomena in different ways" (1978, p. 75). Whereas in the past emphasis has been placed on the aspect of the nursing phenomena most relevant to that particular time and situation, it is apparent from this review of the development of nursing theory that the science of nursing must now take into consideration *all* of the relevant phenomena (Figure 2.7).

Riehl and Roy take the position that many of the current nursing models present a similar view of the human and the environment, and they propose that nursing move toward "a single view of the person and of the goal of nursing," or a unified model (1980, p. 399). If a particular view of the phenomena of nursing science prevails—and I think the work of the nurse-theorist group associated with the National Conference on Classification of Nursing Diagnosis indicates that we are approaching some unity in our way of viewing these major concepts—then we may be entering the first scientific stage of our development.[2] If indeed the development of science proceeds by shifts in the way of viewing phenomena, a unified model will exist

---

[2] The concepts of unitary man, health, and nursing have been addressed by this group which consists of Chairperson Sister Callista Roy, Andrea A. Bircher, Rosemary Ellis, Joyce J. Fitzpatrick, Margaret Hardy, Imogene King, Rose McKay, Margaret A. Newman, Dorothea Orem, Rosemarie Parse, Martha Rogers, Mary Jane Smith, and Gertrude Torres. A report of these proceedings may be found in M. J. Kim and D. A. Moritz (Eds.), *Classification of Nursing Diagnosis: Proceedings of the Third and Fourth National Conferences,* April 1978 and 1980 (New York: McGraw-Hill, 1982), p. 220.

---

for a period of time during which it is useful and eventually will be overthrown by a model which explains the phenomena more completely. What we are looking for are the ideas, or theories, that best fit our observations, but again, we must be cautious and not be limited by observations alone. Remember, that though Copernicus saw the same stars and planets in the sky, he saw them differently from other people. As nursing science develops, we will continue to look at the same major concepts, but at times certain persons among us will see them differently. Theory development in nursing is a continuing revolution.

REFERENCES

Agassi, J. (1968). *The continuing revolution*. New York: McGraw-Hill.

Beckstrand, J. K. (1978). *A conceptual and logical analysis of selected health indicators*. Unpublished Ph.D. dissertation. University of Texas.

Dolan, J. A. (1973). *Nursing in society: A historical perspective*. Philadelphia: Saunders.

Hardy, M. E. (1978). Evaluating nursing theory. In *Theory development: What, why, how?* (pp. 75–86). New York: National League for Nursing Press.

Henderson, V. (1966). *The nature of nursing*. New York: Macmillan.

Johnson, D. (1961). The significance of nursing care. *American Journal of Nursing, 61*(11), 63–66.

King, I. M. (1971). *Toward a theory for nursing*. New York: Wiley.

Kuhn, T. (1970). *The structure of scientific revolutions*. Chicago: University of Chicago Press.

Newman, M. A. (1979). *Theory development in nursing* (pp. 55–67). Philadelphia: Davis.

Nightingale, F. (1946). *Notes on nursing.* Philadelphia: Lippincott. (Facsimile of 1st edition printed in London, 1859).

Orem, D. (1971). *Nursing: Concepts of practice.* New York: McGraw-Hill.

Orlando, I. J. (1961). *The dynamic nurse-patient relationship: Function, process, and principles.* New York: Putnam.

Pelletier, K. R. (1978). *Toward a science of consciousness.* New York: Dell.

Peplau, H. (1952). *Interpersonal relations in nursing.* New York: Putnam.

Polanyi, M. (1962). *Personal knowledge.* New York: Harper Torchbooks.

Popper, K. R. (1965). *Conjectures and refutations.* New York: Harper & Row.

Riehl, J. P., & Sister C. Roy. (1980). A unified model of nursing. In J. P. Riehl & Sister C. Roy (Eds.), *Conceptual models for nursing practice* (pp. 399–403). New York: Appleton-Century-Crofts.

Rogers, M. E. (1970). *An introduction to the theoretical basis of nursing.* Philadelphia: Davis.

Roy, Sister C. (1970). Adaptation: A conceptual framework for nursing. *Nursing Outlook, 18,* 42–45.

Smith, J. (1979). *The idea of health.* Unpublished Ph.D. dissertation. New York University.

CHAPTER THREE

The Focus of the Discipline of Nursing

Margaret A. Newman

A. Marilyn Sime

Sheila A. Corcoran-Perry

A DISCIPLINE IS distinguished by a domain of inquiry that represents a shared belief among its members regarding its reason for being. A discipline can be identified by a focus statement in the form of a simple sentence that specifies the area of study. For example, physiology is the study of the function of living systems; sociology is the study of principles and processes governing human society.

A professional discipline, in addition, is defined by social relevance and value orientations (Donaldson & Crowley, 1978; Johnson, 1974). The focus is derived from a belief and value system about the profession's social commitment, nature of its service, and area of responsibility for knowledge development. These requisites need expression in

Reprinted with permission from *Advances in Nursing Science, 14*(1):1–6, 1991. Copyright © 1991 by Aspen Publishing.

Discussions in the School of Nursing Curriculum Coordinating Committee stimulated ideas for this article. The authors acknowledge the contributions of other members of the committee: Monica Bossenmaier, Dorothy Fairbanks, Carol Reese, Mariah Snyder, and Patricia Tomlinson. The authors also thank Ellen Egan and Kathleen Sodergren for manuscript critiques.

the focus statement. For example, medicine is the study of the diagnosis and treatment of human disease. The social relevance and value orientation of medicine as a professional discipline is conveyed by the commitment to alleviate disease.

Knowledge development within a discipline may proceed from several philosophic and scientific perspectives (worldviews). From this standpoint, the focus of a discipline could be considered paradigm free. The purpose of this article is to present a focus for the discipline of nursing and to discuss the implications of differing paradigmatic perspectives for the nature of nursing knowledge.

CONCEPTS RELEVANT TO THE FOCUS OF NURSING

The focus of nursing as a professional discipline has emerged most prominently over the past decade. A number of concepts have been identified as central to the study of nursing. An example is the frequently cited tetralogy: person, environment, nursing, and health (Fawcett, 1984; Torres & Yura, 1974). While identification of these concepts begins to narrow the focus of nursing, there remains the need for more explicit connectedness and social relevance to describe the field of study that constitutes nursing. Such unconnected concepts do not raise the philosophic issues or scientific questions that stimulate inquiry.

Recently, there has been concentrated emphasis on two concepts as central to nursing: health and caring. Health has been heralded as the centerpiece of nursing knowledge since the days of Florence Nightingale and continues to be discussed by many theorists and researchers (Meleis, 1990; Newman, 1986, 1991; Pender, 1987). The concept of caring also has occupied a prominent position in nursing literature and has been touted as the essence of nursing (Benner &

Wrubel, 1989; Leininger, 1984; Watson, 1985). The accelerated emphasis on health and caring within the past decade has been accentuated by recent Wingspread Conferences (Duffy & Pender, 1987; Stevenson & Tripp-Reimer, 1990) and the devotion of entire issues of nursing scholarly journals to these concepts (*Advances in Nursing Science,* 1981, 1984, 1988, 1990; Nursing Science Quarterly, 1990). These efforts raise questions about nursing's domain of inquiry. Does health or caring represent the focus of the discipline of nursing? Is knowledge gained from research on caring or health specifically identified as nursing knowledge? Although caring and health are indeed central to nursing, no one has developed a unifying focus statement that includes these concepts, and neither concept alone meets the criteria for the focus of a professional discipline. A synthesis of current knowledge development regarding caring and health suggests a focus that meets these criteria.

Caring has generally been linked with the concept of health. In Leininger's historical review of care and caring, she consistently links caring with health and states that "caring is the . . . explanadum for health and well-being (Leininger, 1990, p. 19). Watson combines caring and healing in a causal connection and refers repeatedly to "caring-healing" (Watson, 1988). Benner's tenets, as well, specifically link caring with health and well-being (Benner, 1988).

In a similar fashion, the concept of health is often linked with actions. Pender questions what interventions assist clients in achieving health (Pender, 1990). Newman submits that the essential question of the discipline of nursing "has something to do with how nurses facilitate the health of human beings" and poses the question, "What is the quality of relationship that makes it possible for the nurse and patient to connect in a transforming way?" (Newman, 1990, p. 234).

Further, in nursing, health means *human* health and, most significantly, human health *experience.* Phillips states that "research should focus on . . . the study of people's *experiencing of their health,* their sense of interconnectedness with others, and specifically how health emerges from a mutual process" (emphasis added) (Phillips, 1990). Pender uses the term "health experience" throughout her recent article on health patterns; she points out that "when illness occurs, it is synthesized as part of the on-going *health experience*" (emphasis added) (Pender, 1990, p. 116). Parse has been explicit in her emphasis on human experience as the basis of her theory of man-living-health, (Parse, 1981) which might be rephrased as human health experience.

Considerable evidence exists that caring, health, and health experience are concepts central to the discipline of nursing. These concepts can be related to each other to identify the domain of inquiry for nursing.

A FOCUS STATEMENT FOR NURSING

We submit that nursing is the study of *caring in the human health experience*. This focus integrates into a single statement concepts commonly identified with nursing at the metaparadigm level. This focus implies a social mandate and service identity and specifies a domain for knowledge development. The social mandate and service identity are conveyed by a commitment to caring as a moral imperative. It is important to note that at this level, the concepts are not associated with any particular theory.

The domain of inquiry is caring in the human health experience. This focus dictates that nursing's body of knowledge includes caring and human health experience. A body of knowledge that does not include caring and human health experience is not nursing knowledge. For example, knowledge about health without consideration of caring would be knowledge of a discipline of health. Nursing theories would link caring to the human health experience.

The tasks of nursing inquiry will be to examine and explicate the meaning of caring in the human health experience to ascertain the adequacy of this focus for the discipline, and to examine the philosophic and scientific questions provoked by the focus statement.

DIFFERING PARADIGMATIC PERSPECTIVES

What may appear to be confusing and inconsistent meanings of concepts in the proposed focus may actually be a reflection of the use of different paradigms for knowledge explication (Morse, Solberg, Neander, Bottorff, & Johnson, 1990; Newman, 1990). Nursing research has been conducted from an orientation consistent with at least two, and possibly three, paradigms. Each paradigm specifies a point of view from which the field of study is conceptualized, the assumptions that are inherent in that view, and the basis upon which knowledge claims are accepted. These differing paradigms reflect the shift in focus from physical to social to human science. The three perspectives extant in nursing literature could be described as: particulate-deterministic, interactive-integrative, and unitary-transformative. To explain the effect of a paradigm on the development of nursing knowledge, each perspective will be addressed briefly.

From the particulate-deterministic perspective, phenomena can be viewed as isolatable, reducible entities having definable properties that can be measured. These entities have orderly and predictable connectedness to each other. Change is assumed to be a consequence of antecedent conditions—conditions that, if sufficiently identified and understood, could be used to predict and control change in the phenomena. Relationships within and among entities are viewed as linear and causal. Kinds of knowledge sought include facts and universal laws. Knowledge claims that cannot be refuted are admitted to the body of knowledge. From the perspective of this paradigm, caring in the human health experience could be studied by examining the concepts that comprise the focus. For example, caring could be isolated for study as a human trait having definable and measurable characteristics. Similarly, health could be reduced and dichotomized in terms of characteristics considered healthy versus those considered unhealthy. Caring also could be studied as a therapeutic intervention affecting patients' health in terms of measurable responses (Morse et al., 1990).

From the interactive-integrative perspective (an extension of the particulate-deterministic perspective that takes into account context and experience and legitimized subjective data), phenomena are viewed as having multiple, interrelated parts in relation to a specific context. To explain a phenomenon, the interrelationships of parts and the influence of the context are taken into consideration. Thus, reality is assumed to be multidimensional and contextual. Change in a phenomenon is a function of multiple antecedent factors and probabilistic relationships. Relationships among phenomena may be reciprocal. Knowledge claims may be context dependent and relative. From this perspective, caring in the human health experience would be studied as interactive-integrative phenomena within specific contexts, but still with probabilistic predictability.

The unitary-transformative perspective represents a significant paradigm shift. From this perspective, a phenomenon is viewed as a unitary, self-organizing field embedded in a larger self-organizing field. It is identified by pattern and by interaction with the larger whole. There is interpenetration of fields within fields and diversity within a unified field. Change is unidirectional and unpredictable as systems move through stages of organization and disorganization to more complex organization. Knowledge is personal, involves pattern recognition, and is a function of both viewer and the phenomenon viewed. The subject matter includes thoughts, values, feelings, choices and purpose (Manen, 1990). Inner reality depicts the reality of the whole. From this perspective, caring in the human health experience would be studied as a unitary-transformative process of mutuality and creative unfolding.

RELATIONSHIP OF FOCUS TO PARADIGMATIC PERSPECTIVE

The explication of knowledge relevant to caring in the human health experience is affected by the paradigmatic perspective. As described earlier, concepts in the focus statement could be isolated for study within the first two perspectives, while the unitary-transformative perspective requires the focus to be studied as an indivisible whole. For example, knowledge generated from the particulate-deterministic perspective includes behaviors that characterize caring, physiologic and psychologic aspects of human health, and acontextual rules that relate observable caring behaviors with measurable health outcomes. Examples of knowledge generated from the interactive-integrative perspective include the reciprocal nature of nurse–client interactions, culture-specific caring responses to life process events that are disruptive to health, and rules regarding the influence of specific caring behaviors on the health-related behaviors of particular groups of clients. Knowledge from a unitary-transformative perspective is more difficult to characterize. An example generated from this perspective might be an understanding of the synchrony and mutuality of nurse–client encounters that transcend the time and space limitations of a present situation.

Although multiple perspectives are appropriate for knowledge development in nursing, we are convinced that a unitary-transformative perspective is essential for full explication of the discipline. This position is consistent with a changing world view of the conduct of inquiry into human experience (Bohm, 1980; Briggs & Peat, 1989; Prigogine, 1976) and with other nurse scholars who recognize the value of a unitary perspective to nursing inquiry (Munhall, 1982; Parse, 1981; Rogers, 1970; Sarter, 1988). Insights from our research and practice reveal a rich and fertile glimpse into caring in the human health experience.

The focus of a professional discipline is an area of study defined by the profession's shared social and service commitment. We conclude that the focus of nursing is the study of caring in the human health experience. The explication of nursing knowledge based on this focus takes different forms depending on the perspective of the scientist. We conclude that a unitary perspective is essential for full elaboration of caring in the human health experience. A unified focus derived from the coalescing of theory on caring and health has the potential for claiming the shared vision of nursing.

REFERENCES

Advances in Nursing Science. (1981) *3*(2); (1984) *6*(3); (1988) *11*(1); (1990) *12*(2); (1990) *13*(1).

Benner, P. (1988). *Nursing as a caring profession.* Presented at the meeting of the American Academy of Nursing, October 16, 1988, Kansas City, MO.

Benner, P., & Wrubel, J. (1989). *The primacy of caring.* Menlo Park, CA: Addison-Wesley.

Bohm, D. (1980). *Wholeness and the implicate order.* London: Routledge & Kegan Paul.

Briggs, J., & Peat, F. D. (1989). *Turbulent mirror.* New York: Harper & Row.

Donaldson, S. K., & Crowley, D. M. (1978). The discipline of nursing. *Nursing Outlook, 26*(2), 113–120.

Duffy, M. E., & Pender, N. J., (Eds.). (1987). *Conceptual issues in health promotion. Proceedings of a Wingspread Conference, April 13–15, 1987.* Indianapolis, IN: Sigma Theta Tau.

Fawcett, J. (1984). The metaparadigm of nursing: Present status and future refinements. *Image, 16*(3), 84–87.

Johnson, D. E. (1974). Development of theory: A requisite for nursing as a primary health profession. *Nursing Research, 23*(5), 372–377.

Leininger, M. (Ed.). (1984). *Care: The essence of nursing and health.* Thorofare, NJ: Slack.

Leininger, M. (1990). Historic and epistemologic dimensions of care and caring with future directions. In J. S. Stevenson & T. Tripp-Reimer (Eds.), *Knowledge about care and caring. Proceedings of a Wingspread Conference, February 1–3, 1989.* Kansas City, MO: American Academy of Nursing.

Manen, M. V. (1990). *Researching lived experience: Human science for an action sensitive pedagogy.* Albany: State University of New York Press.

Meleis, A. I. (1990). Being and becoming healthy: The core of nursing knowledge. *Nursing Science Quarterly, 3*(3), 107–114.

Morse, J. M., Solberg, S. M., Neander, W. L., Bottorff, J. L., & Johnson, J. L. (1990). Concepts of caring and caring as a concept. *Advances in Nursing Science, 13*(1), 1–14.

Munhall, P. L. (1982). Nursing philosophy and nursing research: In apposition or opposition? *Nursing Research, 31*(3), 176–177, 181.

Newman, M. A. (1986). *Health as expanding consciousness.* St. Louis, MO: Mosby.

Newman, M. A. (1990). Nursing paradigms and realities. In N. L. Chaska, (Ed.). *The nursing profession: Turning points.* St. Louis, MO: Mosby.

Newman, M. A. (1991). Health conceptualizations and related research. *Annual Review of Nursing Research, 9,* 221–243.

Nursing Science Quarterly. (1990). *3*(3).

Parse, R. R. (1981). *Man-living-health: A theory of nursing.* New York: Wiley.

Pender, N. J. (1987). *Health promotion in nursing practice.* Norwalk, CT: Appleton & Lange.

Pender, N. J. (1990). Expressing health through lifestyle patterns. *Nursing Science Quarterly, 3*(3), 115–122.

Phillips, J. R. (1990). The different views of health. *Nursing Science Quarterly, 3*(3), 103–104.

Prigogine, I. (1976). Order through fluctuation: Self-organization and social system. In E. Jantsch & C. H. Waddington (Eds.), *Evolution and consciousness.* Reading, MA: Addison-Wesley.

Rogers, M. E. (1970). *An introduction to the theoretical basis of nursing.* Philadelphia, PA: F. A. Davis.

Sarter, B. (1988). Philosophical sources of nursing theory. *Nursing Science Quarterly, 1*(2), 52–59.

Stevenson, J. S., & Tripp-Reimer, T., (Eds.). (1990). *Knowledge about care and caring. Proceedings of a Wingspread Conference, February 1–3, 1989.* Kansas City, MO: American Academy of Nursing.

Torres, G., & Yura, H. (1974). *Today's conceptual framework: Its relationship to the curriculum development process.* New York: National League for Nursing Press.

Watson, J. (1985). *Nursing: The philosophy and science of caring.* Boulder, CO: Colorado Associated University Press.

Watson, M. J. (1988). New dimensions of human caring theory. *Nursing Science Quarterly, 1*(4), 175–181.

CHAPTER FOUR

Prevailing Paradigms in Nursing

Margaret A. Newman

THE VARIABILITY AND ambiguity of things called paradigms, both within and outside nursing, have left me at times feeling very confused. In nursing we often refer to the medical paradigm as opposed to the nursing paradigm, or curing versus caring, or health as the absence of disease versus health as an evolving pattern of the whole (Newman, 1986). Parse (1987) has categorized nursing theories in what she has labeled the totality paradigm versus the simultaneity paradigm. Others speak to a quantitative paradigm versus a qualitative paradigm. These perspectives reflect to some degree various philosophies of science. What is the basis for the naming of a paradigm: the discipline it represents, the subject matter it addresses, the thought processes it reflects, dimensions of time-space, the nature of the data collected, or what? One of the international doctoral students at Minnesota asked me why nursing is so caught up in consideration of paradigms. In answer to her question, my thoughts were that it has something to do with the history of the development of nursing science (e.g., our alignment and subsequent disalignment with medicine). When you take a look at the various ways in which we refer to the paradigms, not to mention for the moment the term *metaparadigm,* it is no wonder that graduate students have difficulty sorting it out.

Reprinted with permission from *Nursing Outlook, 40*(1):10–13, 32, 1992.

Adapted from a paper presented at the 1991 National Forum on Doctoral Education, Amelia Island, Fla., June 1991.

Nursing is not alone in having to deal with the paradigm issue. Guba's recent book, *The Paradigm Dialog* (1990), is based on a 1989 conference devoted to this debate in education and related fields. Guba introduced the discussion with an ontologic, epistemologic, and methodologic analysis of four paradigms he identified as relevant: positivism, postpositivism, critical theory, and constructivism. A resume of the basic belief systems associated with these paradigms (Table 4.1) provides a background for sorting out the paradigm issues in nursing.

EXTANT VIEWS IN NURSING RESEARCH

A wide range of beliefs about what constitutes reality and how to go about finding it is reflected in the research taking place in nursing. Sime, Corcoran-Perry, and I have developed our own version of the scientific paradigms we see at work in nursing research (Newman, Sime, & Corcoran-Perry, 1991). We pursued this task for the purpose of delineating how the seemingly disparate work of various members of our faculty can indeed relate to a common focus. We tried not to introduce three new labels, but we did not see our categorizations fitting neatly into those already described. Eventually, rather than referring to them as I, II, and III, we succumbed to assigning descriptive labels to depict the key dimensions in each: I—particulate-deterministic, II—interactive-integrative, and III—unitary-transformative. The idea here is that the first of the paired words describes the view of the entity being studied and the second describes the notion of how change occurs.

From the particulate-deterministic paradigm, which holds closely to the positivist view, phenomena are:

> viewed as isolatable, reducible entities having definable properties that can be measured. These entities have orderly and predictable connectedness to each other. Change is assumed to be a consequence of antecedent conditions—conditions that, if sufficiently identified and understood, could be

Table 4.1 Basic Belief Systems of Positivism, Postpositivism, Critical Theory, and Constructivism

	Ontology	Epistemology	Methodology
Positivism	Realist: Reality exists "out there" Driven by natural laws	Objectivist: Inquirer adopts distant and noninteractive posture	Experimental Empiric Controlled Testing of hypotheses
Postpositivism	Critical realist: Same as positivism except cannot be known because of lack of ability to know	Modified objectivist: Objectivity an ideal that can be only approximated Guarded by critical community	Modified experimental Emphasis on critical "multiplism" (elaborated triangulation)
Critical theory	Critical realist: Reality influenced by societal structures	Subjectivist: Values mediate inquiry Goal is to free participants from effect of ideology	Dialogic, transformative Intended to eliminate false consciousness and facilitate transformation
Constructivism	Relativist: Reality is mental construction, socially and experimentally based Many interpretations possible Multiple realities	Subjectivist: Inquirer and respondent are fused into single entity Findings are creation of process between the two	Hermeneutic, dialectic Aims to identify the variety of constructions that exist and bring them to as much consensus as possible

Excerpted from Guba, E. G. "The Alternative Paradigm Dialog." In E. G. Guba, (Ed.) *The Paradigm Dialog.* Newbury Park, CA: Sage, 1990:17–27.

used to predict and control change in the phenomena. Relationships within and among entities are viewed as linear and causal. (Newman et al., 1991)

From a particulate-deterministic view, only the most objective, observable manifestations of health, such as physiologic parameters, would be considered suitable subject matter for research. A phenomenon such as caring, considered by some as the essence of nursing, either would have to be removed from its context and given an operational definition or would be considered by some as outside the realm of science.

The interactive-integrative paradigm (similar to postpositivism) maintains allegiance to the need for control and predictability in research but views reality as multidimensional and contextual. It acknowledges the importance of experience and includes both subjective and objective phenomena but holds to the objectivity, control, and predictability of the positivist view. It moves away from linearity and acknowledges that in some instances understanding without predictability is enough. Change is viewed as "a function of multiple antecedent factors and probabilistic relationships" (Newman et al., 1991). Knowledge is context dependent and relative. From this perspective, nursing phenomena are viewed as both objective and subjective in reciprocal interaction.

The unitary-transformative paradigm presents a significant shift in the view of reality. The human being is viewed as unitary and evolving as a self-organizing field, embedded in a larger self-organizing field:

> It is identified by pattern and by interaction with the larger whole. . . . Change is unidirectional and unpredictable as systems move through stages of organization and disorganization to more complex organization. Knowledge is personal, involves pattern recognition, and is a function of both viewer and the phenomenon viewed. . . . Inner reality depicts the reality of the whole. (Newman et al., 1991)

Nursing would be studied as a unitary process of mutuality and creative unfolding.

Table 4.2   Shift in Emphasis of Nursing Science

Health focus	Science category	Paradigm
Body ← environment	Biophysical	Single
Body-mind-environment	Biopsychosocial	Multiple
Unitary field	Human*	Emergent

* I now see that from the standpoint of the unitary transformative paradigm, the categorization of nursing science is limiting. The unitary perspective includes the *entire* field—human and beyond—therefore to specify nursing as a human science is inaccurate.

Historically we seem to have moved from addressing primarily the health of the body as affected by environmental factors to interplay of body-mind-environment factors in health, and more recently, to health as an experience of the unitary human field phenomenon embedded in a larger unitary field. These three perspectives, biophysical science, biopsychosocial science, and human science relate to different paradigms. The biophysical sciences are single-paradigm sciences with broad consensus among their members; biopsychosocial sciences involve multiple competing paradigms encompassing both objective and subjective phenomena and relating to different views on the nature of human beings and society (Skrtic, 1990). Human science embraces a view of the human being as a unitary phenomenon and represents a major paradigm shift from the previous two (Table 4.2).

FOCUS OF THE DISCIPLINE

There is another consideration in nursing science. Nursing science is a professional discipline and as such has a commitment to alleviate the problems of society. The nature of the reality we are dealing with must incorporate knowledge of the process of making things better for society—a knowledge of praxis: "thoughtful reflection and action that occurs in synchrony, in the direction of transforming the world" (Wheeler & Chinn, 1989, p. 1).

What is our commitment then? Some would say "the promotion of health." At least two objections to that focus are that (1) it is phrased in the language of intervention and objectivity and therefore excludes the unitary-transformative paradigm; and (2) it is not an exclusive domain of nursing. Others would say "caring." Similar objections might apply: (1) from a positivist view, caring may not be amendable to scientific study; and (2) it is of a universal nature that is not limited to one discipline.

Sime, Corcoran-Perry, and I found that as we progressed in our exploration of prevailing paradigms, our intent became to identify the unifying focus of nursing as a professional discipline. After much discussion among ourselves and other colleagues and review of the literature, particularly over the past decade, we came to the conclusion that the focus of nursing as a professional discipline can be characterized as "caring in the human health experience" (Newman, et al., 1991). This focus synthesizes the phenomena of nursing at the metaparadigm level and makes explicit the nature of the social mandate of nursing. *Caring* designates the nature of the nursing practice participation. *Human health experience* brings together the focus on *human* health and modifies it to mean the human health *experience*. The experiential dimension characterizes the phenomenon as something beyond the traditional objective-subjective perspective. The whole phrase taken together signifies the social mandate to which nursing has responded throughout our history and circumscribes the boundaries of the discipline.

Each major concept of this focus, taken alone, manifests itself in different ways. Morse and her associates (1990) have done a comprehensive review of the variety of ways in which caring has been defined and studied. Their work illustrates the different paradigmatic positions prevalent in nursing today. The same is true for research related to the concept of health. Most of this research emanates from the dominant objective-subjective paradigms (Newman, 1991). At the same time, research that connects caring and the health experience in a mutual, transformative process is emerging as a powerful force within the explication of our discipline.

ARE WE A MULTIPLE-PARADIGM DISCIPLINE?

This question leads to the question of whether the aforementioned focus can be addressed within the objectivist, interventionist tradition. Benner's answer would seem to be "no." Benner (1988) points out that within a social scientific context, caring is "decontextualized" and "operationalized" and becomes just one more therapeutic technique. I take that to mean that this way of viewing caring does not capture the essence of caring.

When Sime, Corcoran-Perry, and I began work on "The Focus of the Discipline" paper, we thought of ourselves as each being representative of one of the three paradigms, but the more we discussed the underlying assumptions of each and came to accept the disciplinary focus of caring in the human health experience, the more each of us became convinced of the necessity of the unitary, transformative paradigm for development of the knowledge of our discipline. We ourselves were transformed in the process. We concluded that knowledge emanating from the first two paradigms is relevant but not sufficient for the full elaboration of nursing science.

Others tend to agree. Pender (1990) describes the shift in nursing to human science, which views persons as unified wholes and focuses on the *experience* of health. She calls for a unitary perspective but still uses the language of objectivity in calling for valid and reliable measures. Parse (1987) says that a discipline encompasses more than one paradigm to guide inquiry, yet clearly takes her stand in what she calls a simultaneity paradigm, one that embraces mutuality and transformation as the nature of human processes.

We seem to be hedging. Are we afraid to give up the certainty in knowing that the positivist view offers? In discussing the movement to new paradigms. Skrtic (1990) points out that the "divorce of science from its contemporary raw empiricist base, and its realliance with judgment, discernment, understanding, and interpretation as necessary elements of the scientific process" means giving up the false certainty of logical positivism and facing the anxiety of less certain forms of knowing.

My original intent was to try to fairly, accurately present each of the prevailing paradigms and to say "Let's agree to disagree and go on about our business." Identifying the paradigms is the easy part. The hard part is acknowledging the pervasive nature of a paradigm, the fact that the values inherent in a paradigm are deeply embedded in the adherents and become normative, indicating what is important and what should be done about it. Paradigms have been compared with cultures in that they represent shared knowledge of what is and what ought to be and *adherents cannot imagine any other way to behave* (Firestone, 1990). This begins to explain some of the uneasiness we experience when an adherent of a paradigm other than our own speaks to the importance of that way of thinking and behaving.

Some argue for accommodation among paradigms; others assert that they have nothing in common. Skrtic (1990) takes the position that "the point is not to accommodate or reconcile the multiple paradigms . . . ; it is to recognize them as unique, historically situated forms of insight; to understand them and their implications; to learn to speak to them and through them. . . ." Moccia (1988) has described the deeper meaning of what is involved in attempts to accommodate different paradigms: the contradiction of trying to control and not to control, the expectation of being able to predict and at the same time acknowledging the process as innovative.

For almost a decade now, thanks to Munhall (1982), we have been aware of the discrepancies between our values as a profession and our practices as scientists. Now it is important to recognize the inconsistencies within our science, inconsistencies we are passing on to students. Lincoln (1990) has experienced the same conflicting values:

> I have often told questioners that research training programs should be two-tracked, with training in conventional and emergent-paradigm inquiry models, followed by training in quantitative and qualitative methods both, completed with computer applications for both quantitative and qualitative data.
>
> But with what I have intuitively come to understand about the pervasiveness of the paradigm we use to conduct inquiry, I now think that training in multiple paradigms (at least in more than a historical sense) is training for schizophrenia. If we want to change new researchers' paradigms, we must do more than legitimate those paradigms in the inquiry outlets, such as journals. We have to train people in them, intensively. We probably ought not to be dividing their attention with other than historical accounts of conventional science. We probably ought to recognize the profound commitments people make to world-views and create centers where such training can go on. . . . (Lincoln, 1990, p. 87)

A movement has begun within nursing education to create centers with a particular focus—perhaps to emphasize one paradigm as dominant. The question is: Are we willing to allow, even encourage, that to occur? Or do we want to give all of the paradigms equal time and emphasis in all the programs? Or perhaps a third alternative might be to promote pockets of parallel emphases from different paradigmatic perspectives within a single program.

Some think that positivism is dead—others see it as alive and well and still dominating the scientific community. In graduate curricula, for instance, is it not true that most "basic" research courses emphasize the tenets of controlled, objective science? Does that not say that this is the way it is and anything else is alternative or deviant? And how many of our courses on theory development begin with the isolation of concepts, development of propositional sets, and derivation of causal relationships? If a faculty seeks to convey a different perspective, they would need to examine their basic ontologic and epistemologic beliefs and develop courses that are consistent with those beliefs.

A PARADIGM SHIFT

Evidence of a paradigm shift exists in nursing. Johnson's bibliometric analysis of nursing literature since 1966 depicts a shift from a scientific medical model to a model based on holism (Johnson, 1990). Sarter's analysis of four contemporary nursing theories reveals commonly shared themes, emphasizing holism, process, and self-transcendence (Sarter, 1988). She suggests that it represents an emerging paradigm. The shift perhaps has not been as revolutionary as Kuhn would have predicted. A recent headline in the *Brain/Mind Bulletin* is apropos: "Can you remember where you were when the paradigm shifted?" (Brain/Mind Bulletin, 1991). Assuming that the shift has occurred, it is incumbent on us to reevaluate the values and structures that shape our discipline.

THE CHALLENGE

The challenge before us is twofold: the need to identify and agree on the central question in nursing, the focus of the discipline, and the need to clarify the scientific values and methods that will address that question.

REFERENCES

Benner, P. (1988). *Nursing as a caring profession.* Paper presented at meeting of the American Academy of Nursing, October 16–18, Kansas City, MO.

Can you remember where you were when the paradigm shifted? (1991). *Brain/Mind Bulletin, 16*(7).

Firestone, W. A. (1990). Accommodation: Toward a paradigm-praxis dialectic. In E. G. Guba (Ed.), *The paradigm dialog* (pp. 105–124). Newbury Park, CA: Sage.

Guba, E. G. (Ed.). (1990). *The paradigm dialog.* Newbury Park, CA: Sage.

Johnson, M. B. (1990). The holistic paradigm in nursing: The diffusion of an innovation. *Research in Nursing and Health, 13,* 129–139.

Lincoln, Y. S. (1990). The making of a constructivist: A remembrance of transformations past. In E. G. Guba (Ed.). *The paradigm dialog* (pp. 67–87). Newbury Park, CA: Sage.

Moccia, P. (1988). A critique of compromise: Beyond the methods debate. *Advances in Nursing Science, 10*(4), 1–9.

Morse, J. M., Solberg, S. M., Neander, W. L., Bottorff, J. L., & Johnson, J. L. (1990). Concepts of caring and caring as a concept. *Advances in Nursing Science, 13*(1), 1–14.

Munhall, P. (1982). Nursing philosophy and nursing research: In apposition or opposition? *Nursing Research, 31*(3), 176–177, 181.

Newman, M. A. (1986). *Health as expanding consciousness.* St. Louis, MO: Mosby.

Newman, M. A. (1991). Health conceptualizations. *Annual Review of Nursing Research, 9,* 221–243.

Newman, M. A., Sime, A. M., & Corcoran-Perry, S. A. (1991). The focus of the discipline of nursing. *Advances in Nursing Science, 14*(1), 1–6.

Parse, R. R. (1987). *Nursing science: Major paradigms, theories, and critiques.* Philadelphia, PA: Saunders.

Pender, N. J. (1990). Expressing health through lifestyle patterns. *Nursing Science Quarterly, 3*(3), 115–122.

Sarter, B. (1988). Philosophic sources of nursing theory. *Nursing Science Quarterly, 1*(2), 52–59.

Skrtic, T. M. (1990). Social accommodation: Toward a dialogical discourse in educational inquiry. In E. G. Guba (Ed.), *The paradigm dialog* (pp. 125–135). Newbury Park, CA: Sage.

Wheeler, C. E., & Chinn, P. L. (1989). *Peace & power: A handbook of feminist process* (2nd ed.). New York: National League for Nursing Press.

PART TWO

Identifying the Pattern of the Whole

When I wrote *Theory Development in Nursing* (1979), I knew there was something missing in the way I was doing research. A student in one of my classes pointed out that measuring an entity at one point in time says little or nothing about the dynamic, evolving phenomena of nursing science. I could see the validity of her point but had no idea as to how we were to remedy the situation. Nevertheless, I jumped into what, for me, was then the unknown and added a chapter calling for more holistic methods (included here as Chapter Five). A major contribution of this chapter was the distinction between dimensions as *reflections* of the whole in contrast to the *additive* perspective of a multivariate analysis. My study of movement and time as indicators of consciousness supported the idea of expanding consciousness across the life span, but the need remained for research consistent with the unitary, transformative nature of the Rogerian paradigm.

A paradigm shift had occurred; yet we were not fully aware of it and continued to pursue research in our usual way. "Nursing paradigms and realities" illustrates how it is possible to embrace one paradigm but try to force it into the methods of another paradigm. Other nursing scientists, particularly Barbara Carper (1978) and Patricia Munhall (1982), began to explicate the different ways of knowing relevant to nursing science and the contradictions between the philosophy of nursing practice and the philosophy of science underlying our research, thereby opening the door for the development of methods consistent with the ontology of our discipline.

A breakthrough came with the realization that the identification of pattern was a way to grasp the whole. The work of the North

American Nursing Diagnosis Association theory task force helped me to see the truth of the maxim: "The whole is different from the sum of its parts." We dealt with thousands of labels of specific problems encountered by nursing practitioners but were unable to come up with a diagnosis of the whole in this way. Sensing of the pattern of the whole (the basis for nursing practice) comes from interaction with the *real persons* who are the clients. The pattern cannot be *constructed* from categorical data.

Step by step, I moved from early research that separated and manipulated the basic concepts to research that sought to identify the pattern of the whole. In the mid to late 1980s, based on my assumption that disease is a manifestation of the pattern of the whole, I embarked on a program of research aimed at pattern identification in persons diagnosed with major disease categories (examples of this research are included in Part Three). This process demanded an understanding of the underlying theory and a commitment on the part of the investigator to be authentic and fully present with the intent to know (to care). In the process of discovering an investigative method appropriate to the paradigm, I discovered that the research was the enactment of practice–research as praxis. Coming full circle, I finally felt that I had arrived at the point of beginning by uniting the theory, research, and practice.

REFERENCES

Carper, B. A. (1978). Fundamental patterns of knowing in nursing. *Advances in Nursing Science,* 1(1):13–23.

Munhall, P. (1982). Nursing philosophy and nursing research: In apposition or opposition? *Nursing Research, 31,*(3), 176–177.

CHAPTER FIVE

Searching for More Holistic Methods of Inquiry

Margaret A. Newman

AS RELATIVE NEWCOMERS to the field of scientific inquiry, nursing researchers have adopted predominantly the methodology of other disciplines in pursuit of nursing knowledge. But just as social scientists have recognized that the methods of physical science could not totally satisfy their needs, so also nursing scientists are discovering that the methods of traditional science may not be sufficient for their needs. It is questionable, for instance, whether or not the phenomena being measured in much of nursing research are really manifestations of wholeness. Furthermore, how can measurement at one point in time (if indeed that is possible) reflect the dynamic nature of the phenomena? As nursing scientists become increasingly sophisticated in methodology and confident in the focus of nursing inquiry, there is a need to develop methods which will depict the holistic, dynamic nature of man as a living system in a constantly changing world. Moreover, there is a need to keep in mind the ultimate purpose of theory development in nursing and to utilize methods which are reflective of the complexity of the real-world situation of practitioner and client.

Reprinted with permission from Newman, M. A. (1979). *Theory Development in Nursing,* (pp. 69–74), F. A. Davis, Philadelphia, PA.

A holistic approach is not to be confused with, or construed to mean, a multivariate approach. It is not the summing up of many factors (psychological, social, physiological, and so on) to make a whole. It is the identification of patterns which are reflective of the whole. What these parameters are will vary according to one's ability to see the whole. For some, the universe can be seen in a grain of sand. For others, characteristics which present identifiable patterns of the individual, e.g., the way a person walks or the way he talks, are a good place to start. The task is not easy. When one has grasped the meaning of holism and identified the phenomenon of inquiry, the next step is to find valid ways of measuring it.

Maslow (1966) has suggested that in the study of human problems we begin with a phenomenological approach. Basic to such an approach is the need for researchers to be astute observers, or as Maslow put it more cogently, "good knowers." In our zeal to obtain valid and reliable research instruments, we may have overlooked the most sensitive of all instruments to measure another human being—ourselves. As we become more knowledgeable about intuition and the powers of our consciousness, we are aware that there is more to knowing than that which we obtain by rational, analytic methods.

Another problem is that much of the research thus far in nursing does not get at intraindividual change, and therefore, can offer no information regarding intraindividual patterns or trends. The majority of the designs have been one-shot comparisons of characteristics within a specific population or cross-sectional designs of a particular characteristic in different age groups. The data are reported in group averages, and, in the case of cross-sectional designs, an assumption must be made that the age groups are from the same population, when we know in reality that there are generational differences. Since, at least at this stage of nursing's knowledge, we need to be able to identify changing intraindividual patterns, it may well be that we will learn more by taking a closer look at fewer cases over time than by looking at many cases at one time. Certainly, much of the research on rhythmic phenomena requires such an approach. As we become clearer as to what phenomena need to be measured and how to measure them, we can then utilize more complex designs which incorporate both longitudinal and cross-sectional testing and thus provide information about intraindividual change in a changing world (Baltes, Reese, & Nesselroade, 1977).

Susman and Evered (1978), scientists in the field of administrative theory, are particularly concerned about the inadequacies of the more traditional, rationalistic methods of science in the development of theories of practice. Their explication of action research as a method for developing theories of practice within living, open systems seems particularly applicable to the need for theories of practice within nursing.

Action research involves the collaboration of the researcher in the real-world situation of the client system with the purposes of improving the situation, developing the competencies of the system, and generating new knowledge. In terms of nursing, the client system would be composed of the nursing practitioner and the client. The purpose of the process would be to improve the health of the client, develop the competencies of the practitioners, and generate new nursing knowledge. The cyclical nature of the process would be the same as that described by Susman and Evered: diagnostic planning, action-taking, data-gathering, evaluative interpreting, and specifying learnings.*

Although the aim of action research is the development of prescriptive-level theory, the method itself is not simply the application and testing of a pre-existing prescriptive solution. It is a continuous collaborative experience with practitioners as the problem is identified and actions are taken to resolve the problem. The situation-problem-action nexus is under continuous revision. Whereas with traditional methods, the problem and solutions are determined in advance and

---

* This segmented sequence, derived from a logical, rational approach, is not consistent with a unitary, transformative approach, which would combine all of these activities at once in an evolving process.

imposed upon a situation, in action research, the researcher begins by being unclear about the situation, problem and actions, and must collaborate with the practitioner and work within a living system. The researcher recognizes that every situation is unique and that the outcome of selected actions cannot be fully known in advance; the process is continuously exploratory in nature.

Susman and Evered assert that action research can make the following contributions to the growth of knowledge:

1. The development of action principles dealing with situational diversity.

2. The development of new kinds of technologies, such as how to diagnose* and how to do something that is *not* prescribed.

3. The development of action competencies—the types of skills needed by practitioners, such as interpretation and judgment skills.

4. The development of the researchers' own competencies of how to act in unprescribed situations.

All of the above outcomes are pertinent to the need in nursing for theories of practice. One further aspect of action research which seems particularly relevant is that it necessitates increased contact and authentic collaboration between the researchers and practitioners. The results of such collaboration should increase the relevance of research to practice and facilitate the application of findings.

Nursing has made considerable progress during the past quarter of a century toward the development of nursing science. We, along with

---

* Diagnose implies a one-way process of observation and evaluation. Substitute "how to facilitate pattern recognition" for the current paradigm in which pattern is an essential feature.

scientists in other disciplines, are on the forefront of exciting new discoveries regarding the development of man and how this relates to health. Scientists from each discipline see these discoveries as an expansion of their own discipline: physicists see it as the expansion of physics, psychologists see it as within their realm, and so on. The same is true regarding the practice which is based on that knowledge. The medical profession sees holistic health as its "rightful heritage," while psychologists have moved ahead in this arena, making contributions of their own. From my standpoint as a nursing scientist, I see the expansion of knowledge related to man's health and the development of practice based on that knowledge as the responsibility, and perhaps the "rightful heritage," of nursing.

We now have a relatively clear concept of the phenomenon of our inquiry. This movement toward a central focus represents, not a unified theory of nursing, but rather an agreement as to what it is we must understand in order to practice nursing. Various conceptual frameworks centered on man as a living system in interaction with a changing environment have emerged, providing the basis for multiple theories regarding health. Nursing theory, then, is theory which describes, [explains, and predicts the patterns of the life process of man which are conducive to health and which prescribe actions to promote these patterns.]* This type of knowledge requires methodologies compatible with the dynamic nature of the phenomena and the complexity of nursing practice.

---

* At this point I had not relinquished the belief that is based on prediction and control of phenomena. I would now substitute "the process of pattern recognition, which illuminates the action potential of the moment" for the bracketed phrases above. See Chapters 3 and 4 for what I consider to be the ontology of the discipline.

REFERENCES

Baltes, P. B., Reese, H. W., & Nesselroade, J. (1977). *Life-span development psychology: Introduction to research method.* Belmont, CA: Wadsworth.

Maslow, A. H. (1966). *The psychology of science.* New York: Harper & Row.

Susman, G. I., & Evered, R. D. (1978). As assessment of the scientific merits of action research. *Administrative Science Quarterly, 23,* 582–603.

CHAPTER SIX

Nursing Paradigms and Realities

Margaret A. Newman

KNOWING WHAT PARADIGM guides one's research is the *key* to findings and, ultimately, to discerning the nature of nursing practice. I would like to share my experience of what happens when one mixes paradigms and different levels of reality.

MAJOR PARADIGMS OF HEALTH

Clarifying one's paradigm is particularly important in regard to the phenomenon of health. There are basically two paradigms of health (Capra, 1982; Ferguson, 1980; Parse, 1981; Watson, 1985). The major and prevailing paradigm is health as the absence of disease. Health as absence of disease varies along a continuum that ranges from high-level wellness at the positive end to the disease state at the negative end. In-between are various stages of adaptation to disease and absence of disease without the extra dimensions implied by the high-level wellness concept. Smith's philosophical study (1981) of the concept of health describes these varying perspectives of health within the absence of disease paradigm. She categorizes the literature about health as clinical, adaptive, role performance, and eudaimonistic. Clinical refers primarily to the medical clinical model and relates

Reprinted with permission from *The Nursing Profession: Turning Points* (pp. 230–235), edited by N. L. Chaska, C. V. Mosby, St. Louis, 1990.

to the absence or presence of symptoms of disease. In terms of the above continuum, it would relate to both disease and absence of disease in terms of prevention (Figure 6.1). The adaptive and role-performance categories are consistent with the stage of adaptation to disease. The eudaimonistic category would be consistent with high-level wellness. The work of a large number of nursing theorists and researchers emanates from this paradigm of health.

The other major paradigm of health is person-centered and encompasses disease as a meaningful aspect of the dynamic pattern of the whole of an evolving person-environment. This paradigm refers to a rhythmic process of increasing complexity. It is a spiraling progression of the unitary person-environment pattern to higher levels of development (Figure 6.2). Martha Rogers (1970) was the first nursing theorist to explicate this paradigm, and a number of other theorists have adopted it as the basis for their work.

So we in nursing find ourselves operating in at least these two major paradigms, and we sometimes get them mixed up. It is possible to do research using the *same* constructs to reflect *different* paradigms—a predicament that leads to misunderstanding and confusion. To maintain communication within our ranks, we need to be clear on our respective paradigms.

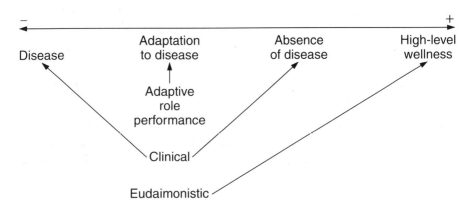

Figure 6.1   Paradigm of Health as the Absence of Disease.

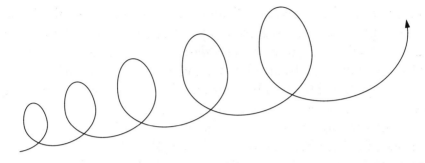

Figure 6.2 Paradigm of Health as a Unitary Evolving Pattern of Person-Environment Interaction.

INFLUENCE OF A PARADIGM ON THE MEANING OF RESEARCH FINDINGS

A paradigm is an overall perspective on things, a worldview. In this case we are talking about a perspective of health. The following accounts illustrate how two different paradigms of health influence the conceptualization and interpretation of similar pieces of research, resulting in findings that are difficult to interpret unless the guiding paradigm is clarified.

My perspective of health fits within the general paradigm of evolving pattern of the whole person-environment. Health is the process of expanding consciousness: all manifestations of life evolving, including disease and disability, reflect this pattern of expanding consciousness (Newman, 1979, 1983, 1986). Consciousness is defined as the capacity of the system (person) to interact with the environment. Movement, time, and space are identified as manifestations of consciousness, that is, the changing pattern of the person's interaction with the environment. Movement and time were operationalized for the purposes of my early research (Newman, 1972, 1976).

Engle (1981) decided to follow up this research with a study of movement and time in elderly women. Her intent, as mine, was to gain a better understanding of how these concepts describe health. She consulted with me regarding operationalization of the concepts and methodological questions and designed her research to test and extend the work I had started. I was eager to participate in a reciprocal exchange of findings and extension of the theory, but after a while I became aware of an uneasy feeling that Engle and I were not talking about the same thing. I was unable to identify the incongruity until she published her research results (Engle, 1984, 1986). Then *her* perspective of health, her paradigm, became clear. Engle's concept of health, as operationalized in her research, is one of functional ability. This measure of health was found to correlate positively with rate of movement, and Engle concluded that speed of movement was an indicator of health. The relevance of this correlation stems from its interpretation in terms of the paradigm of health as the absence of disease. Functional ability would be a measure of role performance within this continuum.

In a paradigm of pattern, which is the foundation for my theory, the viewpoint of more or less healthy is antithetical to the perspective of the paradigm. Health *is* the pattern. Rate of movement is a reflection of the pattern, but it is not a quantification of health. It is not possible within the theory of health as expanding consciousness to conclude that the faster one moves, the healthier one is. The linear, polar notion of more or less ability* is replaced by a notion of pattern.

The communication barrier between Engle and me stemmed from the fact that we were operating from different paradigms of health.

---

* I realize now that my definition of consciousness as "the capacity of the system to interact with the environment" could be interpreted as functional ability within the old paradigm. It does not mean that, in a physical sense. I still support this definition but see it as pertaining to a higher level (frequency) of interaction, sometimes beyond the explicate order.

The operationalization of major concepts in these two research endeavors was the same, but they were being played in two different ballparks, unbeknown, at least for a while, even to the players. Engle was viewing health as more or less functional ability; in that context, faster movement meant healthier. My view of health was an evolving pattern of person-environment interaction (emphasizing the concepts of movement-time-space-consciousness); in that context, faster (or slower) movement helped to describe the total pattern of health.

In another study designed within the context of my general theory of expanding consciousness, the investigators (Nojima et al., 1987) hypothesized that higher consciousness would be related to greater functional ability. Here again the latter variable places the research within an absence of disease paradigm. They found, however, that more disabled persons had higher indices of consciousness than less disabled persons. Rather than representing a rejection of the theory of health as expanding consciousness, as the authors thought, this finding provides data that support a pattern of expanded consciousness in persons whose movement is restricted. It has a completely different interpretation within a paradigm of pattern of the whole person-environment.

These examples are shared to illustrate the difficulties encountered when it is not clear which paradigm guides the conceptualization and interpretation of the research. We have been reared in a society dominated by the absence of disease paradigm. Nurses have sensed intuitively that there is more in the experience of health and illness than the linear, quantitative approach can offer. Sometimes we glimpse the pattern of the whole person-environment for an instant, but then lose that insight, temporarily. There is delight in suddenly seeing the whole pattern and yet confusion because it is not yet grasped entirely. And so we flip back and forth between the two paradigms, perhaps unknowingly. It is like having two jigsaw puzzles cut by the same form but portraying different pictures. The pieces of the two may be interchangeable but meaningless unless they are fit into the picture from which they originated.

LEVELS OF REALITY

Another way in which one's paradigm influences research findings is by specifying what data are acceptable. The paradigm of health as absence of disease is grounded in the scientific method and requires data that are observable and measurable. Such data would be classified in a level of reality referred to as the "see-touch" realm, and perhaps the "behavioral" realm (LeShan & Margenau, 1982). In addition to these realms, LeShan and Margenau (1982) suggest that there are at least three other different constructions of reality: the microcosmic realm, the macrocosmic realm, and the realm of inner experience. Nurses clearly function in the realities of the see-touch realm, the behavioral realm, and the realm of inner experience. The see-touch realm is the most familiar and is quantifiable: pallor, temperature, and pulse are familiar measurements within this realm. The behavioral level is another realm with which nurses are very familiar; this realm includes observations of the way a person talks, what a person chooses to do, who a person relates to, and how a person relates. That too is somewhat quantifiable although the quantities lose some of the meaning in the act. The last realm of reality, that of inner experience, is an important aspect of the health experience; however, phenomena such as joy and sorrow are not quantifiable and cannot be comprehended with see-touch methods. A paradigm that requires observable, "objective" data precludes direct study of the realm of inner experience.

Data from different realms are not contradictory, but each reality has its limits. Different rules apply and therefore observations at one level may not be transferable to another level. Table 6.1 illustrates differences in physical and social reality in terms of the concepts of time and space as suggested by LeShan and Margenau (1982, 157–159).

An example of an attempt to capture one level of reality by measuring another level is seen in studies of time perception. The meaning of subjective time (an inner experience) is limited by measuring it in terms of clock time (a combination of the behavioral and see-touch

Table 6.1 Different Levels of Reality of Time and Space

	Physical Reality	Social Reality
Time	Flows evenly	Flows unevenly
	Past and present causality	Future causality
	Experience as present	Experience of present contains past and future
	Everywhere the same	Differs according to culture and social class
	Clock time	Personal time
Space	Geographical	Behavioral
	Two feet apart	Too close/too far
	Geometric	Personal
	House	Relation to other family members—shared space/private space

realms). The different levels are not contradictory; however, the connection between them is not always apparent. The physical measurement is the "tip of the iceberg" or one arc of a circle. One cannot expect direct correspondence between the part and the whole, *but* the partial information afforded by the physical measurement *is* part of the pattern of the whole person-environment and therefore can be a clue to the pattern.

The intuitive leap that a nurse makes on the basis of very vague, unarticulated information is an example of seeing the pattern of the whole person-environment from partial information. It is the reading of the hologram.* It is allowing that tiny bit of information to project the whole.

---

* The hologram has been widely used as a model that illustrates the phenomenon of information of the whole being imbedded in the part. A fuller discussion of this phenomenon as a model for practice is included in Newman, M. A. (1994), *Health as expanding consciousness* (pp. 104–107), New York, NLN Press.

The different levels of reality are not mutually exclusive, but we sometimes have difficulty communicating across realms. What we comprehend probably depends on our own levels of reality. When I first began to work with the nine dimensions of person-environment interaction that constitutes the framework for nursing diagnosis adopted by the North American Nursing Diagnosis Association (NANDA) (Newman, 1984; Roy et al., 1982), I was aware that my analyses of case study material usually clustered in the categories of exchanging, communicating, and relating. If I could get sufficient data to describe these dimensions of interaction, I could begin to identify their patterns. In retrospect, I see that the levels of reality of these dimensions were more readily observable. At any rate, the pattern of the whole person-environment emerged from partial information. As additional data pertaining to these and other dimensions came forth, of course, the pattern was elaborated and refined.

The nine dimensions of person-environment interaction reflect the three levels of reality described above (Table 6.2). Just to take three nursing practice observations that went into developing the dimensions as examples, one can see how they reflect these different realities. Urinary incontinence, for example, would go into the category of exchanging and is a phenomenon that can be observed and quantified. Abusive behavior would fit into the relating category and is consistent with the definition of behavior as being observable behavior above the reflex level. Low self-concept would fit in the knowing/feeling/valuing categories and is a phenomenon of inner experience. Data from each of these levels of reality are partial reflections of the pattern of the whole person-environment. If these data pertained to one person, the pattern of that whole person-environment would begin to reveal itself.

Since nurses must take into consideration these different levels of reality, either we must be able to switch back and forth between paradigms, or perhaps the paradigm guiding our practice and our investigations must be broad enough to incorporate differing perspectives and methods.

**Table 6.2   Correspondence of NANDA
Dimensions of Person-Environment
Interaction with Levels of Reality**

Levels of Reality	Dimensions of Interaction
See-touch	Exchanging
	Moving
	Perceiving
Behavioral	Choosing
	Communicating
	Relating
Inner experience	Feeling
	Knowing
	Valuing

WHAT ARE THE ESSENTIAL QUESTIONS?

A paradigm of research specifies the kinds of questions that will be asked. We need to ask ourselves, as Rosemary Ellis (Nursing Theory Think Tank Conferences, 1978–1984) asked many times: *What are the essential questions in nursing?*

As I ponder research in other areas, I am struck with some major overriding question that researchers in the field are trying to answer. In biological rhythms, first there was the question of rhythmicity itself— is it a characteristic of all living systems? And all processes within living systems? Then if this is so, where does it come from? Is there an exogenous force or an endogenous clock that maintains the rhythmicity? Volumes of research are devoted to this latter question.

In the area of hemispheric dominance, the question is what are the respective functions of the two cerebral hemispheres. Again, volume after volume of research addresses this basic question and describes the relationship of the two hemispheres in different conceptual terms, as well as the specifics of the various observable functions. The questions engendered by this basic question will keep scientists in the field occupied for many years to come.

The major question in the life sciences is how do new forms of life come into being. This is the question addressed by Sheldrake's hypothesis of morphic resonance* and by Prigogine's theory of dissipative structures.[†] Investigators in laboratories all over the world are pursuing this question.

What then is the guiding, essential question in nursing? The process of theory building is not just an accumulation of facts. It is one powerful, unifying idea evolving. As we become clear on the worldview of nursing, what major question must we answer? I submit it has something to do with how nurses facilitate the health of human beings. The way that the question is asked and the answers that we get, however, depends on which paradigm of health is in place. The question asked by the absence of disease paradigm is: What is the etiology, treatment, and prevention of disease? In the paradigm of health as pattern of the evolving whole person-environment, a question, still focusing on the disease situation, could be: What is the pattern of the whole person-environment depicted by the disease? A further question within a paradigm that depicts nursing as a partnership in the patterning of person-environment development might be: What is the quality of relationship that makes it possible for the nurse and patient to connect in a transforming way?

---

* Sheldrake's hypothesis of morphic resonance states that the characteristic forms and behavior of physical, chemical, and biological systems are determined by invisible organizing fields, referred to as morphogenetic fields, the effect of which is not diminished by space or time and is cumulative. This theory lends an explanation to the observed phenomenon that the difficulty of synthesizing new compounds becomes increasingly easier once the compound has been formed the first time, and this facility is apparent in laboratories great distances from each other (Sheldrake, 1981).

[†] Prigogine's theory of dissipative structures posits that all dynamic systems fluctuate, but rather than averaging out, the process becomes supraordinate to the random perturbations and shifts to a new, higher order, more complex structural form. (Prigogine, I., Allen, P.M., & Herman, R. [1977]).

SUMMARY

We have reached a stage in the development of nursing science when we must be clear about the paradigm that guides our research and must distinguish research relating to one paradigm from that which relates to another. The major prevailing paradigms in nursing today are derived from the prevailing paradigms of health: health as absence of disease, and health as the evolving pattern of person-environment. Research findings will have vastly different meaning depending on which paradigm guides the conceptualization and interpretation. Paradigms determine the research questions to be asked and the data to be sought. A paradigm that integrates different levels of reality would be consistent with the content of nursing practice.

REFERENCES

Capra, F. (1982). *The turning point.* New York: Simon & Schuster.

Engle, V. (1981). A study of the relationship between self-assessment of health, function, personal tempo and time perception in elderly women (Doctoral dissertation, Wayne State University, 1981). *Dissertation Abstracts International, 42*/03B, DEN81-17056.

Engle, V. (1984). Newman's conceptual framework and the measurement of older adults' health. *Advances in Nursing Science, 7,* 24–36.

Engle, V. (1986). The relationship of movement and time to older adults' functional health. *Research in Nursing and Health, 9,* 123–129.

Ferguson, M. (1980). *The aquarian conspiracy: Personal and social transformation in the 1980's.* Los Angeles: J. P. Tarcher.

LeShan, L., & Margenau, H. (1982). *Einstein's space and van Gogh's sky.* New York: Macmillan.

Newman, M. A. (1972). Time estimation in relation to gait tempo. *Perceptual and Motor Skills, 34,* 359–366.

Newman, M. A. (1976). Movement tempo and the experience of time. *Nursing Research, 25,* 273–279.

Newman, M. A. (1979). *Theory development in nursing.* Philadelphia: F. A. Davis.

Newman, M. A. (1983). Newman's health theory. In I. Clements & F. Roberts (Eds.), *Family health: A theoretical approach to nursing care* (pp. 161–175). New York: John Wiley & Sons.

Newman, M. A. (1984). Nursing diagnosis: Looking at the whole. *American Journal of Nursing, 84,* 1496–1499.

Newman, M. A. (1986). *Health as expanding consciousness.* St. Louis: C. V. Mosby.

Nojima, Y., Oda, A., Nishii, H., Fukui, M., Seo, K., & Akiyoshi, H. (1987). Perception of time among Japanese inpatients. *Western Journal of Nursing Research, 9,* 288–300.

Parse, R. R. (1981). *Man-living-health.* New York: John Wiley & Sons.

Prigogine, I., Allen, P. M., & Herman, R. (1977). *Long-term trends and the evolution of complexity.* In E. Laszlo & J. Berman (Eds.), *Goals in a global community: The original background papers for Goals for Mankind* (Vol. 1, pp. 1–63). New York: Pergamon Press.

Rogers, M. E. (1970). *An introduction to the theoretical basis of nursing.* Philadelphia: F. A. Davis.

Roy, C., Rogers, M. E., Fitzpatrick, J. J., Newman, M. A., Orem, D., Feild, L., Stafford, J. J., Weber, S., Rossi, L., & Krekeler, K. (1982). Nursing diagnosis and nursing theory. In M. J. Kim & D. A. Moritz (Eds.), *Classification of nursing diagnoses* (pp. 26–40). St. Louis: C. V. Mosby.

Sheldrake, R. (1981). *A new science of life: The hypothesis of formative causation.* Los Angeles: Tarcher.

Smith, J. (1981). The idea of health: A philosophic inquiry. *Advances in Nursing Science, 3,* 43–50.

Watson, J. (1985). *Nursing: The philosophy and science of caring.* Boulder, CO: Colorado Associated University Press.

CHAPTER SEVEN

Nursing's Emerging Paradigm: The Recognition of Pattern

Margaret A. Newman

IN THE DAYS of Copernicus, about 500 years ago, everyone thought the earth was the center of the universe and that the sun and all the other planets revolved around the earth. From our perspective today that was a very limited view of things. Based on his observations and mathematical calculations, Copernicus said (and people thought he was crazy), that's not the way it is. The sun is the center of things, and the earth and all the other planets revolve around the sun. What a revolutionary idea! Actually, though, it did not change what was there; it just changed the way things were viewed. For one thing, it identi-fied the earth and its inhabitants as simply one aspect of a much larger whole.

We have been involved in a similar revolution. For a long time we thought that disease was the center of our world of nursing. We have a long history of aligning ourselves with medicine in the prevention, treatment and rehabilitation of persons, families and communities in relation to disease. Then, after a century or so of observing that this

Reprinted with permission from *Classification of Nursing Diagnoses* (pp. 53–60), edited by A. M. McLane and published by C. V. Mosby, 1987. Originally titled "Nursing's emerging paradigm: The diagnosis of pattern." Based on paper presented at the Sev-enth Conference on Classification of Nursing Diagnosis, North American Nursing Diagnosis Association, March 9–12, 1986.

approach was not working too well, some people began to say disease is not the center of things, with everything viewed in relation to disease. The whole person, whose nature is indivisible, is the center of things. Disease is simply one aspect of the way a person manifests her- or himself.

Nursing has known this on some level all along, perhaps from the very beginning of our modern history. We have become very familiar with Florence Nightingale's emphasis on health and minimization of the information afforded by disease. She pointed out that pathology teaches us merely the disruptive characteristic of disease, and that understanding of health comes about through observation and experience. Based on observation and experience, she said, nursing can "put the patient in the best condition for nature to act upon him [sic]" (Nightingale, 1859). These words, *observation* and *experience,* have relevance to what we are trying to do today in the development of the concept of nursing diagnosis.

The generating motivations of the founders of this conference on nursing diagnosis, I submit, stem from an intuitive conviction that what nurses were observing and experiencing was different from what medicine was observing and acting upon, and so the movement to identify and elaborate the nursing perspective began in a formal way.

In 1978 the nurse-theorist group invited by NANDA to participate in the development of a classification system for nursing diagnosis met and produced a new way of viewing the phenomena of our practice. Hundreds of observations submitted by the membership of this organization were examined and were clustered into categories according to apparent similarity. At the same time, the group deliberated beliefs about nursing that provided the world view, which in my terms is the paradigm, that structures the perspective from which nursing diagnoses emerge. As in the Copernican revolution, the elements did not change, simply (though it is not simple to accomplish) the way of viewing the elements. The disease and the problems associated with disease were still there, but they were viewed not as entities within themselves but as information about the essential pattern of the person, the human being that is the center of nursing's concern and purpose.

In 1980 Marilyn Ferguson, a recognized spokesperson for new-paradigm thinking, outlined the shift that has taken place in the paradigm of health as we have moved from a paradigm in which disease is the center to a paradigm in which the person is the center. We no longer view disease as totally negative or as an entity unto itself but rather as information about the whole, as a manifestation of pattern. We seek then not to simply eliminate the symptoms of disease but to identify and understand the pattern of which the symptoms are a part. In the old paradigm based on etiology and treatment of disease, the professional is the authority and as such prescribes what the client should do. In the new paradigm based on pattern recognition, the professional is a therapeutic partner and joins with the client in the search for pattern, with its concomitant understanding and impetus for growth.

I think we can have a sense of inner satisfaction that nursing has been at the forefront of knowledge development within the paradigm of pattern. Martha Rogers (1970) emphasized from the outset, in her theory of the unitary nature of human beings, that pattern is the identifying characteristic of a person's wholeness and that the need in nursing practice is to identify *sequential patterns of man's evolving interaction with the environment.*

The point of identifying *sequential* patterns is crucial. The pattern evolves over time. The pattern of relationships that characterized one's childhood, while retaining some essential enduring characteristics, is different from the pattern of the present situation. Each pattern of person–environment interaction is time specific but at the same time contains information enfolded from the past. It is possible to discern the total pattern from the present without reference to the past, therefore, and in a crisis situation, that is probably where one starts. An example related by another nurse (A. Kelly, personal communication, April 20, 1984) illustrates this point:

The client, K., was a young divorced woman who had limited contact with her ex-husband and was not close to her family of origin, even though her mother and her brother lived in the vicinity. She reported feeling bored with her life. She supported herself and her two children, aged two and five, by providing day care for an infant and three other preschool children.

The incident that brought the client to the attention of the nurse was the sudden death of the infant while being cared for at K.'s home. K. responded appropriately, administering CPR and calling the police, but afterward felt guilty and disorganized and overwhelmed by the fighting and turmoil of the children, who had witnessed the event.

Shortly after the infant's death, the nurse telephoned the client offering information about Sudden Infant Death Syndrome (SIDS), and the client asked for help in relating to the children. The nurse visited the home, which was in disarray, and the children were fighting with each other and with the mother. K. was tearful, felt fatigued and wanted to be alone. She had lost interest in her children and was suffering from insomnia. The nurse offered some suggestions regarding the children and invited K. to attend a support group, which she later attended.

The nurse maintained periodic contact with K., and fifteen weeks later, although still sad about the experience of the infant's death, K. had gained considerable comfort from being active in the support group. She took steps to obtain an instructor's license in CPR and had begun teaching a class in it. She helped to present a program about SIDS for day-care providers, arranged to have information about SIDS supplied to each licensed day-care provider and contacted other babysitters who had had similar experiences with SIDS. She volunteered to serve on a local health service board in response to an ad in the newspaper.

At the point when the nurse entered the situation, the client's pattern of interaction was one of disorganization, feelings of sadness and guilt and frustration with child care responsibilities. When the nurse was asked what she saw as her contribution to the situation, she said she thought she provided an organizing force through which the client was able to seek assistance from her mother-in-law for the child care and move out of the home to focus on more outgoing relationships with others in the community. K. developed a close relationship with her mother-in-law for the first time and maintained a friendship with the parents of the infant who died. She was able to allow the children to discuss the experience of the infant's death and to ask questions freely. K. felt as though she had become more outgoing and caring in her relationships with other people.

A diagram of three sequential patterns from K.'s life (see Figure 7.1) illustrates first a relatively closed, low-energy system in which K. existed pretty much alone with her children and the children she took care of during the day. Then the next pattern is one of disruption and disorganization, as K. dealt with the infant's death and subsequently with her feelings and the children's behaviors. The third pattern reflects her reaching out to others to give and receive help. She establishes more intimate relationships with other adults and feels more caring. In comparison, this pattern is characterized by higher energy exchange between K. and her environment and a better quality of relationships.

The identification of the patterns of interaction at these three points in time is simply a reflection of *what is*. It requires very little or no inference or interpretation. It does not imply causality. It is not necessary to know why the client was living a relatively isolated, boring life or why or how it changed in the period following the crisis. From my point of view, this sequence reveals a pattern of expanding consciousness, i.e., a pattern of increased quality and diversity of interaction with the environment. The nurse acted as a source of power, as a pure reference beam which helped the client focus and move beyond herself to relate to others in more caring, meaningful ways.

The role of the nurse within a paradigm of pattern is to help clients recognize their own patterns. A question I have been asked many times is, "But what do you *do about* pattern even if you are able to

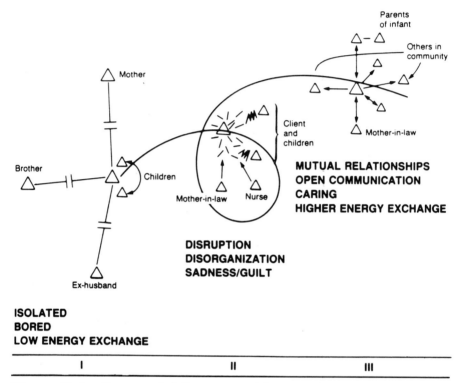

Figure 7.1 Sequential Patterns of Person-Environment Relationships.

identify it?" Nursing diagnosis, in any form, portrays the presenting phenomenon. It pinpoints what you are dealing with. It is a guide to action only insofar as we are knowledgeable about the phenomenon. The isolated phenomena of a problem-oriented paradigm are more familiar to us than the dynamic interactions of a pattern paradigm; so we think we know what to do about them. In this way we delude ourselves into thinking the diagnosis is a guide to specific action.

If diagnosis is not a guide to action, what is it? To focus again on the new paradigm, it is *pattern recognition*. It is the burst of insight that occurs when, suddenly, everything fits together; everything makes sense. And when that happens, the pathway of action opens up. It is like throwing light on a situation. Then one can see clearly and take action. It is different for every situation and therefore cannot be prescribed in advance. It is facilitated by another person's involvement in the interactive process, and that's where nursing comes in.

As I've said before, I think the NANDA health assessment framework based on unitary person-environment patterns of interaction is a step in the direction of helping nurses facilitate patients' pattern recognition (Newman, 1984). I have emphasized that this framework is not a classification system for diagnosis but a guide for assessment, a way of viewing person-environment interaction that focuses on the whole. After seeing the work of the NANDA Taxonomy Committee (March 9–10, 1986), I would propose that the nine patterns of interaction represent one step below the diagnosis level. The diagnosis level would consist of descriptions of the total pattern of the person, a pattern that would reflect the unity of the nine dimensions. This level has not been adequately explicated at this time.

From the previous case study example, Pattern I might be characterized as one of low energy exchange and relative isolation of the person from meaningful adult relationships; Pattern II is one of disorganization, intense, conflictual feelings about herself and her children, and the beginning of an ability to receive support from other adults. Pattern III reveals an increasing number of meaningful mutual adult relationships and more open and caring relationships, which could be considered a modulated, higher exchange of energy. Exploration and elaboration of the nature of the patterns of person-environment interaction have not been undertaken systematically on a large scale: therefore at this time there is little that can be shared with certainty and specificity. I am convinced, however, on the basis of my work with graduate students' explorations and my own pilot work in this area that this unified pattern of the whole is the level at which we function in nursing and is the basis for nursing diagnosis.

As this approach to pattern identification is adopted by nursing practitioners, the skill of sensing into the whole becomes integral to practice. Sensing into the whole is the action component crucial to a paradigm of pattern, and this activity is more one of sensing into oneself than of observing another.

The holographic model of intervention explains this process. A hologram is a form of photography in which the image on the film is formed indirectly by the interaction of light waves being projected from two sources: one from the subject being photographed and one from a pure reference beam such as a laser. The interaction of waves from these two sources forms an interference pattern that reflects the visual image of the subject being photographed. The intriguing aspect of this phenomenon is that every portion of the resulting holographic film contains information about the whole! If a small corner of the film is torn off and a light is projected through that segment, the image portrayed will be the entire image originally photographed, not an arm or a leg as would have been the case if one had torn a segment from the film of a conventional photograph.

This model for the way things work has been used to explain the way the brain works (Pribram, 1971) and even the way the universe works (Bohm, 1980). And more to the point in terms of our present concern, it has been used to explain the process of therapeutic interaction.

It helps to imagine the phenomenon of interference patterns to visualize a rock being thrown into a lake. As it hits the water, a series of circular waves emanate from the point of impact and spread outward. Then imagine another rock being thrown into the water nearby with its own pattern of expanding waves. Within seconds the two wavefronts will reach each other and interact, forming a new pattern, an interference pattern (see Figure 7.2). Eventually the interference pattern expands to replace the original two patterns, which have become *one pattern containing information about the whole of both.*

Now imagine two persons interacting in place of the two rocks (see Figure 7.3). The waves that emanate from each person interact with the

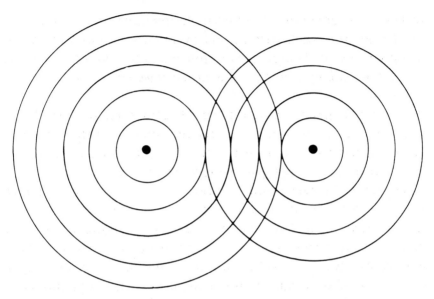

Figure 7.2 Formation of an Interference Pattern.

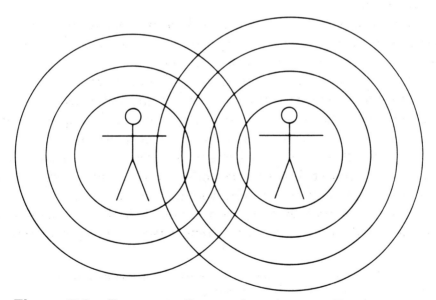

Figure 7.3 Person-to-Person Interference Pattern.

waves of the other person, forming an interference pattern that contains information from each pattern and eventually becomes the whole. One's own pattern (being) contains information about the whole. *The way to get in touch with the pattern of the other person is to sense into one's own pattern.*

Just as in holography a pure reference beam is used to depict the picture of the subject, in therapeutic relationships it is helpful to try to clear one's field to act as a mirror of the client's pattern and thereby facilitate that client's own pattern recognition.

The goal of this type of intervention (which is really nonintervention) is not so much that we as professionals identify the pattern of the client but that clients have the experience of recognizing their own patterns of interacting with the environment. It is characteristic of the process, however, that the professional will have a similar experience. This kind of insight occurs suddenly, as when a picture comes into focus and one sees clearly, or knows thoroughly (the meaning of diagnosis).* Through this heightened understanding the pathway of action unfolds.

So what does this mean for the work of this conference? I think it means that the key to nursing diagnosis lies not so much in information outside ourselves (i.e., data *about* the client) as it does in information that is continuously available to us within our pattern of interaction with the client. This insight can occur instantly and is just as readily available to a nurse in the rapid pace of an acute care setting as it is for someone who has time for more deliberate contemplation.

For some, this approach appears to be rejecting the information that we have collected thus far. For others, it is totally subjective, not objective, and therefore not valid from their perspective.

To these charges I say first that it does include the information of the old paradigm but from a different perspective, the perspective

---

* The word diagnosis comes from the Greek words for *knowing* and for *through* or *thoroughly* and literally means *knowing thoroughly.*

of what that information means in terms of the total pattern of energy exchange. I agree that it is not objective, because in a paradigm of pattern things are no longer separated into subject and object. There are no separating boundaries between what is outside (objective) and what is inside (subjective), and so neither is it subjective.

A paradigm of pattern eliminates dichotomies. In a holographic model, we have access to the total information of our world through ourselves. By offering ourselves as windows of the world we can facilitate this insight, "knowing thoroughly," in others.

In the past decade, a rapidly increasing number of nurses have endorsed the concept of pattern as central to nursing diagnosis and action (Benner & Wrubel, 1982; Bramwell, 1984; Crawford, 1982; Fitzpatrick, 1983; Newman, 1979, 1983; Parse, 1981). The need now is to get on with it! When the uncertainties and doubts arise as we are faced with letting go of the safety of the old and taking the leap to the new, it's tempting to want to hold back. But as Marilyn Ferguson (1983) has said, "If you keep acting like you've always acted, you're going to get what you've always got." I am convinced that we in nursing want more for ourselves and for the patients we serve. We want the authenticity and meaning and satisfaction that comes when our relationships with patients have made a difference. Each of us has experienced the coherence of such moments from time to time and we want to be able to explicate that knowledge of the whole to others. As we are able to do this, we can have confidence that our practice derives from a nursing paradigm.

REFERENCES

Benner, P., & Wrubel, J. (1982). Skilled clinical knowledge: The value of perceptual awareness, I and II. *Journal of Nursing Administration,* *5,* 42; *6,* 28.

Bohm, D. (1980). *Wholeness and the implicate order.* London: Rout-ledge & Kegan Paul.

Bramwell, L. (1984). Use of the life history in pattern identification and health promotion. *Advances in Nursing Science, 7,* 37.

Crawford, G. (1982). The concept of pattern in nursing: Conceptual development and measurement, *Advances in Nursing Science, 5,* 1.

Ferguson, M. (1980). *The aquarian conspiracy: Personal and social trans-formation in the 1980s* (pp. 1–6). Los Angeles: J. P. Tarcher.

Ferguson, M. (1983). *Conference: Power of knowing.* Minneapolis.

Fitzpatrick, J. J. (1983). A life perspective rhythm model. In J. J. Fitz-patrick & A. L. Whall (Eds.), *Conceptual models of nursing.* Bowie, MD: Brady.

Newman, M. A. (1979). *Theory development in nursing.* Philadelphia: F. A. Davis.

Newman, M. A. (1983). Editorial. *Advances in Nursing Science, 5,* x.

Newman, M. A. (1984). Nursing diagnosis: Looking at the whole. *American Journal of Nursing, 84,* 1496.

Nightingale, F. (1859 Facsimile). *Notes on nursing: What it is, and what it is not.* Philadelphia: J. B. Lippincott.

Parse, R. R. (1981). *Man-living-health: A theory of nursing.* New York: Wiley.

Pribram, K. (1971). *Languages of the brain.* Belmont, CA: Brooks, Cole.

Rogers, M. E. (1970). *An introduction to the theoretical basis of nursing.* Philadelphia: F. A. Davis.

CHAPTER EIGHT

Patterning

Margaret A. Newman, PhD, RN, FAAN

THE ASSUMPTION OF holism, considered basic to nursing practice, calls for an understanding of the whole, knowledge of the total system in interaction with the environment. Some people think that knowledge of the whole is impossible, that science just does not work that way. The way to gain this understanding, they say, is to attain knowledge of the parts and gradually build knowledge of the whole. That has not worked very well for knowledge in a practice discipline. Summing up the parts just does not make a whole. We are left with fragmented knowledge that is not very helpful in practice.

Part of the problem is our belief that our theories offer true knowledge of reality. We conscientiously sort out the elements of a theory and begin to treat these similarities and differences as though they have a separate existence. The physicist David Bohm (1980, p. 7), suggests that "We will thus be led to the illusion that the world is actually constituted of separate fragments and . . . this will cause us to act in such a way that we do in fact produce the very fragmentation implied in our attitude to the theory."

When confronted with the maxim that the whole must be grasped in order for the parts to be meaningful, many clinicians will respond

Excerpts reprinted with permission from *Conceptual Issues in Health Promotion,* (pp. 36–48), Report of Proceedings of a Wingspread Conference, edited by M.E. Duffy & N.J. Pender, April 13–15, 1987. Indianapolis: Sigma Theta Tau International.

that wholeness is only an ideal; the reality of the situation, they say, is seen in the form of an irregular pulse, an obstructed artery, a malignant tumor, a paralyzed limb. Bohm asserts that wholeness is what is real and that what is observed is limited by fragmentary thought. The problem is the way we look at things, not the things in themselves. As we become aware of our fragmentary thought and move beyond it, our approach to reality (the patient, health) will be whole, and then the response will be whole.

So it has seemed reasonable to me to move in the other direction: to start searching for the whole. There are certain characteristics of people that constitute patterns that identify the whole. Things such as the way a person moves, or talks, or at the microscopic level, the genetic pattern. These are enduring characteristics that identify a person across the life span. The question is how to utilize these dimensions as reflections of the whole. The task is not one of fitting together pieces of a puzzle but of seeing these dimensions as *sketches* of the whole. As one's vision improves, the picture of the whole will have greater clarity and detail, as when a projected image comes into focus.

Bohm (1980) has theorized that there is an underlying pattern of the whole (meaning the whole universe). This pattern, which he calls the implicate order, is unseen but becomes manifest in the explicate order, the things we can see, feel or hear. The assumption that I make is that *whatever* manifests itself in a person's life is the explication of the underlying implicate pattern and that the phenomenon we call health is the manifestation of that evolving pattern. Disease, if it is present, is viewed not as a separate entity but as information about the essential pattern of the person in interaction with the environment.

The pattern is self-organizing over time, meaning it is becoming more highly organized with more information. With increasing information, there is increasing capacity to interact with the environment. The pattern of relationships that characterized one's childhood, while enduring in some essential ways, is different from the pattern at later stages of development. Each pattern is time specific *and* contains information which is enfolded from the past and which will unfold in the future.

In my attempts to describe the overall pattern of a person, I am comforted by Gregory Bateson's (1979) assertion that as of 1979 there was *no conventional way* of explaining or describing the phenomenon of human interaction. That statement was made within the context of Bateson's concern about "the pattern which connects" (p. 12), a kind of metapattern, which I would equate with Bohm's implicate order. Bateson makes some points that I find helpful in understanding pattern and is adamant that it cannot be understood by simple measures of quantity: "It is impossible, in principle, to explain any pattern by invoking a single quantity. But note that *a ratio between two quantities* is already the beginning of pattern" (p. 58). Bateson regards the difference between *number* and quantity as profound. He regards number as being in the same world of thought as pattern. The way to recognize number is to count, and counting is a form of pattern recognition and is discontinuous. Quantity, on the other hand, is continuous and belongs in the world of analogic and probabilistic computation.

To illustrate that pattern and quantity are different logical types, Bateson suggests imagining an island with two mountains on it. When the ocean rises (a quantitative change), the island may become two islands. The qualitative pattern was latent before the quantity effected a change. When the change occurred, it was sudden and discontinuous. This example reminds me of situations in which the qualitative pattern of, say, a disease is latent, and then some quantitative change occurs, and the disease pattern manifests itself in a sudden and discontinuous event.

Pattern recognition comes from within the observer—which means that with any set of data or sequence of events, an infinite number of patterns are possible. If someone offers you the sequence of numbers— 2, 4, 6, 8—you will more than likely perceive a pattern of even numbers and predict that the next number will be 10. However the pattern might be 2, 4, 6, 8, 11, 13, 15, 17, 20, 22, 24, 26 and so on. You are the one perceiving the pattern and the pattern will be changed by new information, or by anything that forces a new perception of it, like a change in context. For example, a behavior means one thing at age 5 and another at age 25. The nature of this phenomenon is such that the pattern cannot be predicted *with certainty* because the additional information has not happened yet (Bateson, 1979, p. 31).

Back to my attempts to describe pattern. At first, using the NANDA dimensions of person-environment interaction derived from nursing clinicians' observations, I collected as much data as possible about a particular individual and tried to synthesize a whole pattern (Newman, 1984). Although this approach was helpful in forcing attention on the dynamic, interactive nature of all of the phenomena all at once, it was obvious that the pattern changed over time and it was confusing to try to make all of the information explicate at the same time. The pattern was unfolding in time. Then a colleague presented data about a patient in her caseload, and as we discussed the pattern of the person, it became apparent that it must be portrayed as sequential patterns over time. This is, as a matter of fact, what Martha Rogers (1970) exhorted us to do almost two decades ago. This particular case involved a crisis event and the portrayal of the changing pattern included at least three time frames: prior to the crisis event, immediately following the crisis event, and 15 weeks post-crisis. This analysis was helpful in understanding the unfolding pattern. (See example described in Chapter 7.)

The next step was to use this approach to analyze data from interviews of 'healthy' adults. Subjects were asked to think back over their lives and describe the most meaningful persons or events. After the data were organized into sequential patterns, a follow-up interview was conducted to share the investigators' diagrams with the subjects to seek their validation or revision of the projected pattern (Newman, Vail, & Cowling, 1986). The current stage of this research has been to follow this protocol to interview patients who have coronary artery disease or cancer.

Case Study

An example from a study of persons with coronary heart disease (see Chapter 12) illustrates the process.

From our interviews with J. we learned that as a child he was one of six brothers and two sisters. He said that nothing was ever given to him; if he wanted something, he had to earn the money and buy it. He learned early to be self-supporting. He said he was always a loner, that he was never interested in being with a gang, or crowd. His mother impressed upon him the need to find a job, something that he would like, because he would have to work the rest of his life. Finding and succeeding in a job became the predominant theme of his life, one that was often thwarted. He said he had had over 38 different jobs. Eventually he was able to work his way up the ranks in his job as a mechanic and became the top mechanic in his company. He felt as though he had achieved his goal regarding his job and was very proud of this achievement, but he later lost his job after his second heart attack and triple bypass surgery.

He got married when he was in his early 20s, was married for 12 years and had two children, a son and a daughter. Marriage, to him, was all work and no play. During this period he said he never showed his anger. He felt obligated to help where help was needed, e.g., children, senior citizens.

After his divorce, he started to enjoy life more and became active in community affairs and the Moose Lodge. He became the hospital visitor for the Lodge and in this capacity came in contact with sickness and death. He regarded that time as one of comradeship and friendship. He became head of the Lodge and got to know a lot of people across the state and felt that he received a lot of respect. A businessman who was the Lodge secretary was particularly helpful to him. That same year he had two coronary artery surgeries and a third heart attack.

Right now he feels as though he has no goal or does not know what his goal in life is. He has no job. He has a live-in girlfriend who has been supportive, but he feels as though he does not have anything (in terms of money) to offer her and this bothers him. He says he wants a steady job but does not know what to go for.

He considered volunteering for a job taking care of an island because it would afford him time alone to think things through such as: When is the big one going to come? How are his kids going to take it? How is his lady friend going to react? He wonders what it would be like to be gone, or perhaps reincarnated as a free spirit. He said he never talked to his girlfriend about these things, that he never talks to her about anything important. In comparing his attitude now to his previous burden of work and unexpressed anger, he says that he has developed a more mellow attitude, one that lets life come as it comes.

A diagram of the sequential patterns in this man's life begins with him as a loner within a large family (see Figure 8.1). His mother impressed him with the need to find a good job. There is no mention of his father. The medical record indicated his father was an alcoholic. In the second pattern, he is married and is going from one job to the next trying to find the perfect job and eventually achieving his goal. This period seems to be one of drudgery—"all work, no play"—and unexpressiveness. Then he and his wife were divorced and he began to enter into new relationships in the community and with a number of women friends. His most meaningful interactions during that time were within the context of his Lodge; he mentioned the secretary of the Lodge in particular as being very helpful to him. He was involved increasingly in helping others. It was during this period that he had several heart attacks and three episodes of coronary artery surgery.

Now in the present pattern, he expresses a great deal of doubt regarding the direction of his life. He is facing death and wants to think things out. He daydreams of dying, being reincarnated and coming back as a "free spirit." An overall view of his pattern over time is one of moving from isolation and minimum interaction to a tremendous drive to find the perfect job, to expanding interaction with friends and

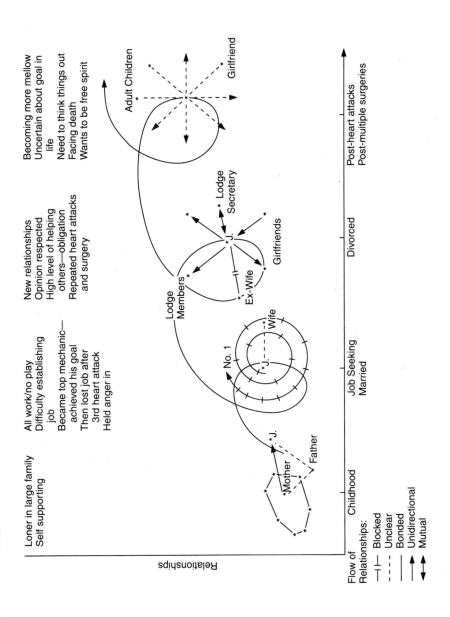

Figure 8.1 Critical Periods—Case Study of J.

community associates, and lastly a desire to transcend his physical state and become a free spirit.

What do these patterns mean in terms of health? I think the most pressing need, regardless of the clients' disease status, is their relationship with other people. The task that each of them is facing is to engage in meaningful, reciprocal relationships. They want to be able to talk about things that are important to them, to express a full range of emotions and to be truly themselves, but in many instances they do not know how. They want to let go of the drive to accomplish, to win, to be best.

A flippant answer to the question of what patterns are health generating would be: Be born into the right family, one in which there are caring human relationships that facilitate self-expression. Since we cannot mandate that for everyone, not even ourselves, we can start where we are. For me that means helping clients get in touch with their pattern of interacting and the insight that accompanies it—the phenomenon of pattern recognition.

Sometimes it is difficult to see the pattern of evolving consciousness in the present moment, but it will unfold over time. Even when the pattern appears to be disorganized or blocked, the direction of its unfolding is a higher level of consciousness. This means that when viewed within the larger pattern, the direction is up, even when it's down. Bateson (1979) comments that we have a hard time realizing that "whatever the ups and downs of the detail within our limited experience, the larger whole is primarily beautiful" (p. 19).

The aspect of patterning that I have not addressed is the relationship between macroscopic patterns of interaction and microscopic patterning of the individual. Some recent work at the National Institutes of Health supports a holistic view from the 'hard' sciences. Candace Pert (1986), a biochemist, refers to the 'bodymind' as a single integrated entity. She regards neuropeptides and their receptors as an *information network* within the body and interprets her findings as demonstrating the consciousness of the body. Bernard Engel (1986) depicts circulation as behavior, which he defines as an *integrated* set of responses. He emphasizes the functional significance of behavior within a particular context at a specific time. Based on the assumption that these internal behavioral manifestations are explications of an underlying pattern of consciousness, the next step is to try to make the connections between the external and internal levels of reality.

Fundamental aspects of pattern, regardless of the perspective, include connectedness, context and time. As we concentrate on looking for the whole, the larger pattern will emerge.

REFERENCES

Bateson, G. (1979). *Mind and nature: A necessary unity.* Toronto: Bantam.

Bohm, D. (1980). *Wholeness and the implicate order.* London: Routledge & Kegan Paul.

Engel, B. T. (1986). An essay on the circulation as behavior. *The Behavioral and Brain Sciences, 9,* 285–318.

Newman, M. A. (1984). Nursing diagnosis: looking at the whole. *American Journal of Nursing, 84,* 1496–1499.

Newman, M. A. (1986). *Health as expanding consciousness.* St. Louis: Mosby.

Newman, M. A., Vail, J. D., & Cowling, W. R. (1986). *Interview protocol: pattern of person-environment interaction.* Unpublished manuscript.

Pert, C. B. (1986). The wisdom of the receptors: neuropeptides, the emotions, and bodymind. *Advances, 3,*(3), 8–16.

Rogers, M. E. (1970). *An introduction to the theoretical basis of nursing.* Philadelphia: F. A. Davis.

PART THREE

Transforming the Meaning of Health and Practice

The paradigm of nursing science introduced by Martha Rogers' conceptual framework demanded a new concept of health. The health-illness continuum prevalent in the 1960s and 1970s maintained a dichotomous view of health and illness. It did not meet the criterion of wholeness specified in the new paradigm. I knew from personal experience that health encompassed disease. Suddenly, extrapolating from the theory of biological rhythms, I saw health and illness as one unitary process evolving rhythmically through order and disorder. And Itzhak Bentov's explanations of how life is evolving to higher, more inclusive consciousness helped me bring together a concept of health as the evolving pattern of the whole—a pattern of expanding consciousness. The assumption that consciousness is coextensive in the universe is inclusive: It applies not only to individuals, but also to families and communities.

Basic to this point of view is an understanding of pattern. In pursuit of a method to identify pattern, I applied an experiential dialectical approach. It quickly became apparent that the researcher and the researched were involved in a dynamic, mutual process of expanding consciousness.

There is a need for much further development of this approach. Some of the work on the life patterns of persons with major disease manifestations is included to illustrate the development of theory and practice within this new concept of health. Sensing into the pattern of the whole, so essential to pattern recognition, is difficult to explicate. A beginning attempt to do so has been made in "The Spirit of Nursing."

CHAPTER NINE

Toward a Theory of Health

Margaret A. Newman

CURRENT CONCEPTUAL MODELS in nursing emphasize the focus of
the nursing process, i.e., the phenomenon of man, or the interactive
component, which facilitates that process. Although most nursing theorists recognize health as the goal of nursing, the terms used to define
health are often broad and general and are subject to multiple inter-
pretations. A precise conceptualization of the nature of health is required in order to specify theory which relates to that phenomenon.

Most would agree that health is *not* the absence of disease, or complete psychological and social well-being, for these states are nonex-
istent in the complexity of our changing world. Some progress was
made in an understanding of health when health and illness were
placed on a continuum. This conceptualization recognizes the dynamic, changing relationships portraying different degrees of health
and illness; however, it still maintains the dichotomy between the two
by polarizing health at one end of the continuum and illness at the
other end. If the goal of nursing is to move the individual toward
health, then in this context, that means *away* from illness. In so doing,
the dichotomy is maintained.

Reprinted with permission from Newman, M. A. (1979). *Theory Development in
Nursing* (pp. 55–67), F. A. Davis, Philadelphia. Based on paper presented at the Nurse
Educator Conference, New York City, December 1978.

What is needed is a synthesis of the concepts of health and illness. This view is based on Hegel's dialectical process of the fusion of opposites: one state of being unites with its opposite and brings forth a synthesis of the two. Applying this process to health and illness, there is, on the one hand, a condition specified as disease and, on the other hand, its opposite, which will be called non-disease. The fusion of the two antithetical concepts brings forth a synthesis, which can be regarded as health.

Disease—Non-disease → Health

When health is viewed as the synthesis of disease and non-disease, the following statements can be considered as basic assumptions:

1. *Health encompasses conditions heretofore described as illness, or in medical terms, pathology.*

   A person who has a pathological condition is not necessarily "ill." Experience with persons incapacitated in various ways by chronic disease reveals that, for the most part, these people do not consider themselves sick. They may be unable to walk or to care for themselves, but from their point of view, they are *not* sick, unless perhaps they are inconvenienced by the common cold. As a matter of fact, nearly everyone of adult age has some condition which could be specified as pathological, with varying degrees of incapacitation, but each person is still very much a whole person.

2. *These "pathological" conditions can be considered a manifestation of the total pattern of the individual.*

   This statement is based on Rogers' prior assumption that "Pattern and organization identify man and reflect his innovative wholeness" (1970, p. 65). The pattern which is manifested in disease may be regarded as a clue to what is going on in the person's life, the dynamics of which the person may be unaware of and cannot communicate in any other way.

3. *The pattern of the individual that eventually manifests itself as pathology is primary and exists prior to structural or functional changes.*

   An illustration of this point may be seen in Bahnson and Bahnson's (1966) theory regarding the rhythms of cancer. They maintain that the person who develops cancer manifests a pattern of very controlled interaction with the environment and very uncontrolled or chaotic internal processes; another way of describing it would be as rigid external rhythms and disorganized internal rhythms. If this theory holds, the pattern exists prior to the development of the cancer; the cancer is simply a manifestation of the pattern.

4. *Removal of the pathology in itself will not change the pattern of the individual.*

   This principle can be seen in the previous example regarding cancer. The pattern of which the cancer is a manifestation is a total pattern of the person. Removal of the cancer will not change the basic pattern. As Western medicine has begun to seek holistic approaches, practitioners are beginning to recognize that disease is not something "to be gotten rid of," but something to be understood and experienced and regarded as a teacher or message. Disease can be regarded as an integrating factor, and as such, it is important in the evolutionary process of the individual, and not something to be squelched.

5. *If becoming "ill" is the only way an individual's pattern can manifest itself, then that is health for that person.*

   Illness, as an integrating factor, may accomplish for the person what he was unable to do otherwise. Stone (1978), a Jungian psychologist who has embraced a holistic approach to health and illness, points out that in his practice he "doesn't keep track of people getting well anymore." Not that he is not pleased when someone does "get well," and not that feeling well is an unimportant consideration, but it is not of such importance that it is sought to the exclusion of the higher purpose of integration of self, which then frees energy for an expanding consciousness.

6. *Health is the expansion of consciousness.*

Health is viewed as the totality of the life process, which is evolving toward expanded consciousness. Man represents one stage of this evolution. The direction of evolution within the individual person as well as within the species of mankind is toward expansion of awareness to greater dimensions.

CONCEPTUAL FRAMEWORK

Based on this synthesized view of health, what are the basic concepts the interrelations of which describe the process? Any attempt to identify and understand the basic components of such a process might be considered a presumptuous endeavor. Capra (1975) a physicist, points out that a current hypothesis in physics "not only denies the existence of fundamental constituents of matter, but accepts no fundamental entities whatsoever—no fundamental laws, equations, or principles." Such a position, however, does not preclude an attempt to understand the total by an examination of selected phenomena. He continues:

Physicists have come to see that all their theories of natural phenomena, including the 'laws' they describe, are creations of the human mind; properties of our conceptual map of reality, rather than reality itself. The conceptual scheme is necessarily limited and approximate, as are all the scientific theories and 'laws of nature' it contains. All natural phenomena are ultimately interconnected, and in order to explain any one of them we need to understand all the others, which is obviously impossible. What makes science so successful is the discovery that approximations are possible. If one is satisfied with an approximate 'understanding' of nature, one can describe selected groups of phenomena in this way, neglecting other phenomena which are less relevant. Thus one can explain many phenomena in terms of a few, and consequently understand different aspects of nature in an approximate way without having to understand everything at once.

That is the intent in this conceptual framework: to understand many phenomena, the phenomena of the life process, and therefore of health, in terms of a few. The concepts which constitute this framework are movement, time, space, and consciousness (Figure 9.1). The postulated interrelationships of these concepts are as follows:

1. Time and space have a complementary relationship.

2. Movement is a means whereby space and time become a reality.

3. Movement is a reflection of consciousness.

4. Time is a function of movement.

5. Time is a measure of consciousness.

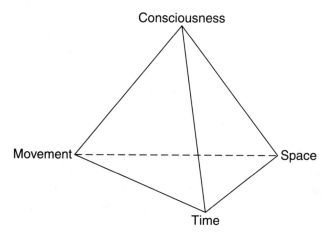

Figure 9.1 The Conceptual Framework.

Life, as we know it, is composed of the energy of matter and motion, and each may be transformed into the other. The energy of motion is transformed into the energy of mass, and vice versa. At the sub-atomic level, particles have no meaning as isolated entities but only as interconnections of things. The world, then, according to Capra (1975), must be viewed as a complicated network of interrelated changing events, as dynamic patterns of activity, with space aspects and time aspects.

The complementarity of space and time can be seen at different levels of analysis. At the level of macrocosmic systems there is the likelihood of antimatter galaxies where time flows in the opposite direction from our perspective, and "black holes" in space where time and space are "wrapped up" by gravitation in unimaginable ways; at the microcosmic level, subatomic particles of matter appear to be going backward in time (Pelletier, 1978). The complementarity of space and time can also be seen in everyday events. The highly mobile individual lives in a world of expanded space and compartmentalized time. When one's life space is decreased, as by either physical or social immobility, one's time is increased. Such a situation can be an opportunity for attention to the space that is within. As one is able to transcend the limitation of three-dimensional space, the experience of time changes and with it the level of consciousness. The concept of space, then, is inextricably linked to the concept of time. There is reason to believe that the nature of the relationship which is being described at the macrocosmic and microcosmic levels will hold also at the humanistic level as the concepts of life space, personal space, and inner space are examined in relation to time.

Movement is an essential property of matter. Movement brings about change, without which there is no manifest reality. The reality of our world is manifest in the change occurring between two states of rest (Bentov, 1978). This action-rest cycle is evident at the micro level in nerve action spikes and complex muscular rhythms, and at the macro level in the pattern of body movements, breathing rhythms, and interactive patterns of life activities. Illustrating this action–rest cycle, the pattern of body movement contains the necessary rhythm of preparation, action, and recovery (Hall & Cobey, 1974).

Within this general pattern, the body movement of each person is specific to that person. Each individual naturally adopts a walking tempo which is most efficient in energy expenditure for that person (Ralston, 1958). The total pattern of movement appears to be reflective of the organization or disorganization of the thought and feeling processes of the individual. Disharmony in the body-world system is reflected in disharmony of body movements. Where there is excess tension, this leads to alienation of the affected parts of the body, and there is loss of versatility of potential action. Action requires internal organization as well as clarity of organization of the corresponding world structure. Changes in either internal organization or perception of external organization will be reflected in the pattern of movement (Hall & Cobey, 1974).

Movement is seen, then, as an awareness of self. Awareness of self is closely connected with awareness of the body. Kinesthetic awareness is viewed by some as the "basic process of knowing which subtends all bodily actions, and synthesizes them" (Mickunas, 1974). Further it is considered to be the basic perceptual organ of space and time as it contains memory of the past and expectations of the future. For instance, when we become angry or hurt, these feelings are reflected in our muscles and may remain there unless released through aggressive action. The muscles become a kind of storehouse for locked energies. In addition, our world space is changed each time we make a move; the objects of the world are perceived in terms of their potential movements, or the possibilities for action (Hall & Cobey, 1974).

Movement is a means of communicating. We express ourselves in movement and gesture. This expression of self in movement is refined in the body arts, but occurs more generally on a day-to-day basis. Language itself requires a rhythm of muscular activity, which consists of successive waves of patterned movements. This rhythm is shared by the listener. The harmony of the movement-speech configuration of the speaker is reflected in the muscular patterns of the listener, provided that they are relating: "This mutual dance facilitates an empathic understanding of the other person's world through complementary movements" (Hall & Cobey, 1974). The rhythm and pattern which are reflected in movement are an indication of the internal organization of the person and his perception of the world. Movement provides a means of communication beyond that which language can convey.

Movement relates also to the experience of time. The illusiveness of time has been a mystery which has intrigued philosophers for centuries. Einstein's theory of relativity brought the relativity and subjectivity of the time experience under scrutiny by the scientific community, and subsequently scientists in nearly every field have sought to describe and understand the meaning of time. Piaget (1966), in his studies of both children and adults, led the way in postulating time as a function of movement. This relationship is supported by my previous research, e.g., when an individual is forced to walk at a rate which is slower than his preferred rate of walking (normal tempo), his perception of time changes (Newman, 1976). The slower one walks, the faster the objective time of the world seems to be passing. (This relationship seems to be modified by the individual's awareness of the movement activity, as described in the previous chapter.)

In addition to the relationship between movement and time, an even more intriguing association seems to be emerging from these data: a relationship between age and time. On the surface, this relationship appears to contradict the movement-time nexus; since from a number of standpoints, the older person appears to be slowing down. If this were true, extrapolating from the movement-time relationship, one would anticipate that time would be perceived as passing faster. The opposite appears to be true on preliminary testing; another explanation is needed.

Bentov (1977) has postulated that time is a measure of consciousness. He calculates an index of consciousness by establishing a ratio of subjective time (the number of seconds judged to have elapsed) to objective time (actual clock time). For example, if one thinks 4 seconds have elapsed, but according to the clock, only 1 second has elapsed, the ratio would be 4/1 with a resulting index of consciousness of 4 (as compared to a ratio of $1/1 = 1$). When this index is applied to the data from my previous research (Newman, 1976), it reveals the following trend:

Age (Means)	Time Subjective/ Objective		Consciousness Index
23(N = 52)	40/43	=	.93
28(N = 90)	40/31	=	1.29
71(N = 23)	40/17	=	2.35

With increasing age, the index of consciousness increases. These data are consistent with the position that the direction of the life process is toward expansion of consciousness.

In recent years, studies of the brain have made us aware that there are dimensions of consciousness which have been neglected and, to some extent, have not been easily available to us. The major hemisphere, usually the left, is primarily responsible for the analytical, sequence-perceiving processes, while the minor hemisphere, usually the right, is primarily responsible for the synthesis-oriented, symbolic and intuitive modes. The scientific and technological values of our Western society have emphasized the rational, logical processes to the neglect of intuitive, holistic processes. This emphasis has been reinforced developmentally, in that processing in one hemisphere inhibits processes in the other (Fischer & Rhead, 1974). With the recognition that the products of logical rational approaches are not necessarily desirable, we have begun to recognize the need for the development and facilitation of the intuitive processes. We have available to us a realm of consciousness which many of us are not utilizing. This situation can be likened to tuning in to a small AM radio rather than a refined stereophonic system. The possibility exists for us to tune in to higher frequencies. The human range of frequency response extends into the astral realm. According to Bentov (1977), the fact that some human beings are able to perceive at the higher end of this range explains the experiences of so-called paranormal, or psychic, phenomena. The direction of the evolution of life is toward higher and greater frequency of energy exchange.

As the process of evolution takes place, we must be prepared for, and recognize in others, jumps in consciousness beyond our present capacities. Scholars from a variety of disciplines are in agreement that there is no matter devoid of consciousness and that consciousness is co-extensive (Watson, 1978; Capra, 1978; Muses, 1978). The higher the level of consciousness, the more the interpenetration of energy fields, and with this interpenetration, evolutionary jumps occur. According to Bentov (1978), you "catch it [expanded consciousness] like you catch the flu." Watson (1978) illustrates this point with an example from studies of monkey colonies on a small island adjacent to the southernmost island of Japan. In 1952 the winter was particularly severe, and the monkeys were given supplementary feedings of sweet potatoes. There was a problem, however, with the containers for the food, and the potatoes fell out and became coated with sand, which made it difficult for the monkeys to eat them. One day a young female monkey took her sweet potato to a nearby freshwater stream and washed it. According to Watson, such an innovation in the monkey world was "tantamount to inventing the wheel." This young monkey then taught her mother and her siblings and her other monkey friends how to wash the potatoes. Very slowly the knowledge spread through the community of monkeys. Six years passed, and in March 1957, a significant number of monkeys, perhaps 99 in all, had learned to wash potatoes. Then the hundredth monkey learned the trick, and 20 minutes later every monkey in the community was doing it! By that evening monkeys on two neighboring islands, with no physical contact, were washing sweet potatoes! The knowledge had reached a kind of critical threshold, or critical mass, beyond which it became common knowledge.

SUMMARY

The expansion of consciousness is what life, and therefore health, is all about. Movement, time, and space have been selected as correlates of developing consciousness and means whereby we can gain some understanding of the process. This framework provides a view of health as the totality of life process and therefore one which encompasses disease as a meaningful aspect. In this context, the goal of nursing is not to make people well, or to prevent their getting sick, but to assist people to utilize the power that is within them as they evolve toward higher levels of consciousness.

REFERENCES

Bahnson, C. B., & Bahnson, M. B. (1966). Role of the ego defenses: denial and repression in the etiology of malignant neoplasm. *Annals of the New York Academy of Science,* 125(3):827–845.

Bentov, I. (1977). *Stalking the wild pendulum.* New York: Dutton.

Bentov, I. (1978). *The mechanics of consciousness.* Paper presented at symposium on New Dimensions of Consciousness, sponsored by Sufi Order in the West, New York.

Capra, F. (1975). *The tao of physics.* Boulder, CO: Shambhala.

Capra, F. (1978). *The tao of physics.* Paper presented at symposium on New Dimensions of Consciousness, sponsored by Sufi Order in the West, New York.

Fischer, R., & Rhead, J. (1974). The logical and the intuitive. *Main Currents,* 31(2):50–54.

Hall, R. L., & Cobey, V. E. (1974). The world of crystallized movement. *Main Currents,* 31(1):4–7.

Mickunas, A. (1974). The primacy of movement. *Main Currents,* 31(1):8–12.

Muses, C. (1978). *Higher dimensions and systems relating science and spirit.* Paper presented at symposium on New Dimensions of Consciousness, sponsored by Sufi Order in the West, New York.

Newman, M. A. (1976). Movement tempo and the experience of time. *Nursing Research,* 25:273–279.

Pelletier, K. R. (1978). *Toward a science of consciousness.* New York: Dell.

Piaget, J. (1966). Time perception in children. In Fraser, J. T. (ed.), *The Voices of Time* (pp. 202–216). New York: George Braziller.

Ralston, J. H. (1958). Energy-speed relation and optimal speed during level walking. *Int. Z. Angewandte Physiol. Einsch. Arbeitsphysiol.,* 17:277.

Rogers, M. E. (1970). *An introduction to the theoretical basis of nursing.* Philadelphia: F. A. Davis.

Stone, H. (1978). *Holism: A new vision of man, a new vision of health.* Paper presented at conference on Holistic Perspectives: A Renaissance in Medicine and Health Care. Philadelphia.

Watson, L. (1978). *Evolution and the unconscious.* Paper presented at symposium on New Dimensions of Consciousness, sponsored by Sufi Order in the West, New York.

CHAPTER TEN

Health as Expanding Consciousness Applied to Families

Margaret A. Newman

WAYS OF DEFINING health in families are parallel to the general views of health—absence of disease, functional capacity, normality, and high-level wellness (Offer & Sabshin, 1966, as cited in Beavers, 1977). The first, absence of disease, is a negative way of defining health: If a family has a member who is emotionally ill*, it is not healthy; if it does not have anyone so defined, it is healthy. The second classification relates to optimal functioning of the family. Optimal functioning is defined by whatever theoretical system is being used. A third way of looking at health is in terms of normality. A "normal" family would be the "average" family and fall somewhere in the middle between functioning well and nonfunctioning. And last, a fourth definition of health has to do with the process of growing and changing

---

Reprinted by permission of John Wiley & Sons, Inc., copyright © 1983. Excerpted from Newman, M.A. (1983). Newman's health theory. In Clements, I., & Roberts, F. (Eds.), *Family Health: A Theoretical Approach to Nursing Care* (pp. 161–175). New York: Wiley.

* I would add "physical" illnesses as well as "emotional" even though from my point of view they are not separated.

as essential to "getting and staying" healthy and calls forth the idea of optimal functioning, or well-being.

My theory of health, which is based on a synthesis of disease and nondisease, is relevant to family health. Beavers (1977, p. 123) describes the fantasy of family health:

> . . . professionals develop a fantasy of health for individuals and families that is derived from observing disturbed people, and they carry this definition in their heads as an ideal, with few supporting data. The usual . . . professional will stoutly deny that his family of origin was normal, and he has great doubts about the health of his friends' families! We are not unlike energetic and enthusiastic missionaries who encourage others to be good Christians, but have knowledge only of sinners. Perhaps many of us, like wise missionaries, recognize that the fantasy is just that, a construct, possibly useful to urge ourselves and others toward a laudable but eternally unattainable goal. If we do not recognize the abstract quality of the fantasy of health, our work with struggling individuals can be discouraging.

I contend that my synthesized view of health recognizes the fantasy of health as described by Beavers and substitutes instead the reality of fluctuating patterns of energy exchange (sometimes seen as disease) that are part of the developing consciousness of the family and of the individual members of the family. Within this framework, the basic assumptions of my original theory can be restated in terms of families:

1. *Health encompasses family situations in which one or more family members may be diagnosed as ill.* The family that is frequently referred to in the literature as "ill" is the *schizophrenogenic family*. This term refers to certain patterns of family interaction that are associated with a schizophrenic offspring (Beavers, 1977). Minuchin's work has expanded the idea of illness of children as a function of the family pattern to illnesses with physiological manifestations, such as anorexia nervosa and diabetes (Minuchin, Rossman, & Baker, 1978). The "ill" individual is an integral part of the family system.

2. *The illness of family member(s) can be considered a manifestation of the pattern of the family interaction.* The child who becomes schizophrenic has somehow been targeted to assuage the pain of an unresolved parental conflict (Beavers, 1977). The child with anorexia nervosa is often found in a family with an enmeshed pattern of interaction: in such a family the boundaries between family members are not clear (Minuchin et al., 1978). Other illnesses are being investigated in terms of their relationship to the overall family pattern.

3. *Elimination of the disease condition in the identified ill family member will not change the overall pattern of the family.* The preceding family situations illustrate situations in which the family dynamics work for the system at the expense of one member. In some situations, when one member changes his or her behavior, another will assume that role (Swanson, 1981). For instance, in a situation of psuedomutuality between parents in terms of power and control, the woman may be absorbing the conflict. Everything appears to be running smoothly for years until some time later, she becomes depressed. As the woman becomes stronger and begins to be more assertive in expressing her needs, another member of the family, most likely one of the children, may assume the role of peacemaker, "swallow" the conflict, and, perhaps, begin to develop stomach aches.

4. *If one person's becoming ill is the only way the family can become conscious of its pattern, then that is health (in process) for that family.* In the situation described above, as long as no one becomes ill, the family appears to be functioning well. The depression of the mother is a signal, which, if explored in terms of the family system, could throw light on the pattern of family interaction. The symptom (in this case, depression) is not an isolated incident to be viewed as an entity in and of itself but rather as a manifestation of the pattern of interaction of the family. As the members

of the family begin to recognize their participation in the pattern, they are able to vary their responses to each other.

5. *Health is the expansion of consciousness of the family.* Consciousness has been defined previously as the informational capacity of the system, a factor that can be observed in the quantity and quality of responses to stimuli. This definition applies to family as well. As the quantity and quality of responses of family members increases, there is more spontaneity within the family. Members are no longer locked into limited responses, and growth can occur. In a rather extensive study on family structure. Pratt (1976) concluded that higher interaction within the family and between the family and the community was associated with health; she referred to this type of family as the energized family.

The major concepts of this theory of health—movement, time, space, and consciousness—may be applied to the dynamics of family systems. Kantor and Lehr (1975) have identified space and time as two of the dimensions whereby family members accomplish their goals of affect, power, and meaning. Although they do not identify movement as one of the concepts of their framework, it is inherent in the concept of power. According to these family theorists, "Power relations focus on the aspects of freedom and restraint within family organization . . ." and can be quantified "by the degree of freedom or restraint in members' *movements*" (italics mine) (p. 49). The concept of consciousness is apparent in their conceptualization of meaning. They view the family as a complex informational field and assert that self-knowledge of the system or subsystem and the ability to represent oneself accurately to others is the primary target of the meaning dimension.

The space dimensions that are important in the family include not only the physical space of the family dwelling but also the maneuverable spaces defined by territoriality, the ways in which family members distance themselves from each other and from the world outside the family and those spaces that family members are willing to share. Time within the family is analogous to space, in that there is private time of family members, shared time, and coordinated time. These variations in the way family members spend their time take on a rhythm of family interactions consisting of work time and play time, and in these ways family members determine their boundaries and distances in terms of time as well as space.

Movement is apparent in the movement of individuals in and out of the family and the degrees of freedom of individual movement. The importance of this dimension becomes accentuated when one family member is restricted in movement by physical paralysis. That person no longer has the option, without considerable assistance, to move about from private space to shared space or from private time to shared time. His control over his life space-time is greatly diminished. The physical limitations of one family member influence the movement-space-time freedom of another member. Other family systems place value constraints on individual movement in and out of the family system.

A comparison of the dimensions of the major concepts of this theory as they relate to individuals and families is seen in Table 10.1.

NURSING IMPLICATIONS

Nursing's goal is to facilitate the health of the family. Within this theoretical framework, health of the family is the expansion of consciousness of the family. Translating this concept into action means facilitating the development of an increased range of responses of family members to each other and to the world outside the family. In addition, it means facilitating the refinement, or quality, of those responses.

Table 10.1 Individual and Family Dimensions Related to Major Concepts of Newman's Theory of Health

	Movement	Time	Space	Consciousness
Individual	Personal tempo Muscle memory Coordination of body movement Preparation-action-recovery cycle Nonverbal communication	Subjective time Time perspective Use of time	Personal space Inner space Life space	Informational capacity of the person Self-knowledge and ability to communicate self Quantity* and quality of personal responses to stimuli
Family	Coordinated movement of language between speaker and listener Coordinated movement of dancing, love-making, sports Freedom of individual movement within system Movement outside of family	Private time Coordinated time Shared time	Territoriality Shared space Distancing	Informational capacity of the system Quantity* and quality of interaction within family Quantity* and quality of interaction with community

* Substitute "diversity."

The first task is to assess the health of the family in terms of the major concepts of the theory—movement, space, time, and consciousness. Obviously family participation in the identification of these patterns is essential, since it is their consciousness, not that of the nurse, that is the purpose of the activity. One might begin to identify:

- The pattern of movement within and outside the family.
- Coordination of space and time.
- Quantity and quality of interaction within family.
- Quantity and quality of interaction between family and community.

The pattern that will emerge will be one of energy flow and will illustrate areas where energy is blocked, areas where energy is depleted or diffuse, or areas where there is buildup, or overload. As the overall pattern of family emerges, the informational capacity of the family will be increased by participation in this process of pattern identification.

SUMMARY

This theory of health equates health with the life process and the life process with expanding consciousness. *Consciousness* is defined as the informational capacity of the living system, a capacity that manifests itself in the quantity* and quality of responses of the system to its environment. A framework for studying consciousness has been set forth with emphasis on the concepts of movement, time, and space. Basic to this approach to health is a view of disease as a reflection of the pattern

---

* Substitute "diversity."

of man-environment interaction and as possibly an integrating factor that provides the tension necessary for expanding consciousness. Health, then, is not a utopian state to be achieved and maintained but rather the process of living to be experienced as fully as possible.

The application of this theory of health to families extends the definition of consciousness to the consciousness of the family system. Based on the assumption of expanding consciousness, the interactive pattern of the family is viewed as a manifestation of expanding consciousness. If the interaction takes the form of disease in one or more family members, then that can be used to examine the pattern and facilitate the development of a greater response repertoire for the persons involved. Health of the family is viewed as a process of expanding consciousness.

REFERENCES

Beavers, W. (1977). *Psychotherapy and growth—A family systems perspective.* New York: Brunner/Mazel.

Kantor, D., & Lehr, W. (1975). *Inside the family—Toward a theory of family process.* New York: Harper Colophon Books.

Minuchin, S., Rossman, B., & Baker, L. (1966). *Psychosomatic families—Anorexia nervosa in context.* Cambridge: Harvard University Press.

Offer, D., & Sabshin, M. (1978). *Normality.* New York: Basic Books.

Pratt, L. (1976). *Family structure and effective health behavior—The energized family.* Boston: Houghton Mifflin.

Swanson, A. (September 7, 1981). Personal communication.

CHAPTER ELEVEN

Newman's Theory of Health as Praxis

Margaret A. Newman

A FUNNY THING happened on the way to developing a method to examine expanding consciousness. In the process, we (Newman, Vail, & Cowling, unpublished pilot study, 1985) discovered that sharing our perception of the person's pattern with the person was meaningful to the participants and stimulated new insights regarding their lives. We discovered that our participation in the process made a difference in our own lives. We suspected that what we were doing in the name of research was nursing practice. And it was fun! Research was really fun. It was no longer the monotony of repeating the same procedure 80-odd times to meet statistical inference conditions. It was no longer acting as a robot-like manipulator of subjects' (objects) behavior. It was participating in an authentic way with real people and attending to meaningful events in their lives in a way that transformed both the researcher and the researched.

These revelations may not seem spectacular to those who have been socialized in experiential methods of inquiry, but to an old experimentalist, these discoveries were indeed significant. I even wrote a poem (of sorts) about it.

Reprinted with permission from *Nursing Science Quarterly,* 3(1):37–41, 1990.

I don't like
Controlling, manipulating
Other people.

I don't like
Deceiving, withholding
Or 'treating'
People as 'subjects' (objects).

I don't like
Acting as an 'objective'
Nonperson.

I do like
Interacting
Authentically: listening, understanding,
     communicating
Freely.

I do like
Knowing and expressing myself
In mutual
Relationships.

Circa 1985

The purpose of this article is to present an overview of my theory of health as expanding consciousness (Newman, 1979, 1983, 1986), the emerging research methodology, and its relevance to nursing practice; but first I would like to describe the steps that brought me to a reconciliation of my research with the theory.

I have come full circle. My earliest investigation (Newman, 1966) was based on individualized, reciprocal interaction with hospitalized patients; it incorporated my own thoughts and feelings as a factor that made a difference in the findings. The original intent of the study was to identify needs of patients (content), but in the process of doing so, the more significant finding was the process used in identifying the needs. That particular research contributed directly to the knowledge of nursing practice, and it was also personally meaningful to me as the investigator and to the patients who participated as subjects.

Later my imagination was captured by the games-like intrigue of the scientific method. I was challenged to convert holistic parameters of a person's living experience into manipulable artifacts in the laboratory in an attempt to test some very basic relationships of movement-time-consciousness (Newman, 1972, 1976). The outcomes of this research were tangential to the meaningful experiences that were their source. The aspect of the research that stimulated insight regarding the relevance to nursing practice was the debriefing interviews in which I earnestly sought a greater understanding of the person's experience in movement-time-consciousness. Buoyed by Bentov's conceptualization of time as an index of consciousness (Bentov, 1978), I continued to pursue this line of investigation in an attempt to demonstrate the expansion of consciousness with age (Newman, 1982; Newman & Gaudiano, 1984), but the inability to adequately capture the major variables or to rule out intervening variables raised questions regarding the validity of the methods to test the theory and pointed toward other modes of inquiry.

Gradually I moved around the circle. With the help of colleagues and graduate students I began to explicate a method of inquiry that was consistent with my theoretical assumptions, that is, the open, interactive nature of the evolving pattern. Early in my career as a naive researcher with no particular external expectations regarding my work, I stumbled onto the conclusion that the important part of my research was the process involved in interacting with patients. The process was the content. Then in response to the scientific norms of the day, I separated process from content (or at least I thought I did) and even enjoyed using process to manipulate content. Now I have again come to the realization that, in nursing in particular, the process *is* the content.

Reinharz (1983) calls for knowledge that explains the transformation from one point to another. In the case of the theory of health as expanding consciousness, the question is: What is the process by which expanding consciousness occurs? Morgan (1983) too points out that we need to get beyond the idea that knowledge is somehow *foundational,* or like solid building blocks. He equates the quest for knowledge with human practice:

> . . . when we engage in research action, thought, and interpretation, we are not simply involved in instrumental processes geared to the acquisition of knowledge but in *processes through which we actually make and remake ourselves as human beings* (p. 373) (emphasis added).

Lather (1986) has captured the essence of what we experienced in the process of identifying pattern: research as praxis—research which involves the researched in a process of inquiry characterized by negotiation, reciprocity, and empowerment. *Lather sees a priori theory as central to praxis-oriented research:*

> For praxis to be possible, not only must theory illuminate the lived experiences . . . it must also be illuminated by their [the researched] struggles. Theory adequate to the task of changing the world must be open-ended, nondogmatic, informing, and grounded in the circumstances of everyday life: . . . (p. 262)

This insistence on the necessity of a priori theory renders a strictly interpretive, phenomenological approach inadequate. Lather insists that there must be an intersection between people's self-understanding and the researcher's theoretical stance, which seeks to provide a change-enhancing context:

> Data must be allowed to generate propositions in a dialectical manner that permits use of a priori theoretical frameworks, but which keeps a particular framework from becoming the container into which the data must be poured. The search is for theory which grows out of context-embedded data . . . (p. 267)

Even though she sees reciprocity between the researcher and the researched as providing better data, Lather asserts that this purpose (outcome) is not enough and urges researchers to use the research to help participants understand and change their situations. This is what research on health as expanding consciousness is all about.

OVERVIEW OF THE THEORY OF HEALTH AS EXPANDING CONSCIOUSNESS

My theory of health as expanding consciousness stems from Rogers' theory of unitary human beings (Rogers, 1970). Rogers' assumptions regarding the patterning of persons in interaction with the environment are basic to my view that consciousness is a manifestation of an evolving pattern of person-environment interaction. The way in which I define consciousness is important to an understanding of the theory. This concept of consciousness is defined as the informational capacity of the system (in this case, the human being); that is, the ability of the system to interact with the environment. Consciousness includes not only the cognitive and affective awareness we normally associate with consciousness, but also the interconnectedness of the entire living system, which includes physiochemical maintenance and growth processes as well as the immune system. This pattern of information is part of a larger, undivided pattern of an expanding universe.

Rogers' insistence that health and illness are simply manifestations of the rhythmic fluctuations of the life process led me to view health and illness as a unitary process moving through variations in order-disorder. From this standpoint, one could no longer think of health and illness in the dichotomous way characterized by the medical paradigm; that is, health as absence of disease or health as a continuum from wellness to illness. Health and the evolving pattern of consciousness are the same.

A person is identified by her or his pattern, which is evolving through various permutations of order and disorder, including what in everyday language is called health and disease. The process is one of increasing complexity. Both what we call health and what we call disease are manifestations of the evolving pattern.

Bohm's theory of reality as undivided wholeness supports this view. Bohm (1980) posits an unseen, underlying pattern as the primary order of reality; he calls this the implicate order. All the tangible things of the world, the things we can see and hear and feel, are explications of the implicate order; the explicate order is secondary to the implicate order. Disease (and all other observable manifestations of human functioning) can be seen then as the explication of an underlying pattern. From this perspective, disease is considered a manifestation of the wholeness of the underlying pattern, not a separate entity.

A view of health as the evolving pattern of the whole requires a non-fragmentary world view. To illustrate the fragmentary nature of our usual perspective, Bohm suggests that one imagine the view of a fish tank through two television cameras. The camera projections, coming from different angles, contain images of the fish and flora that are clearly related, in movement, timing and space relations. Each projection portrays a valid picture of the contents of the fish tank but neither portrays the whole picture. The projections are different points of view of the same larger reality, *just as disease and absence of disease are different points of view of a much larger reality.* They cannot be separated from the whole, except in our fragmentary way of viewing them.

In the process of identifying pattern, it is important to remember that the implicate order cannot be made explicit all at once, but is present in various stages of enfoldment and unfoldment (Bohm, 1980). The pattern of interaction which represents the current pattern of a person's life incorporates information enfolded from the past and information which will unfold in the future. The pattern takes on new meaning when viewed in relation to previous patterns and presents an opportunity for new action (transformation).

The situation that brings a person to the attention of a nurse represents a time in people's lives when the old rules don't work anymore, a time when one must make a choice. The task is to learn how things work, to discover the new rules, and to move on to a new level of being, understanding. Both Bateson (1979) and Young (1976) see this task as the purpose of life. I see it as the crux of the situations in which nursing can assist people in their search for understanding of the evolving pattern of their lives.

Young (1976) sees human beings as coming into this world from a state of *potential freedom* and moving through several stages of loss of degrees of freedom in the descent into a deterministic (physical) world. The first stage he calls the stage of *binding*. In this stage one is bound into the larger network of the whole in which everything is regulated and the individual is sacrificed for the good of the whole. There is very little individual identity or choice here. The next stage, *centering*, is the one in which the individual establishes some sort of identity and self-consciousness and self-determination. In this stage the self breaks with the authority of the first stage. This is a competitive, persuasive stage in which one seeks to gain power over others and gain power for oneself. The turning point is the stage of *choice*. In this stage the things that worked in the past don't work anymore. What was formerly considered progress is no longer progress. It is in this stage that the task is to learn the new rules. There is a realization of self-limitation that precedes the reformation (transformation) that makes it possible to begin the journey back to freedom by going beyond oneself into the stages of *decentering* and *unbinding*.

A parallel between my theory of health as expanding consciousness and Young's theory of evolution (see Figure 11.1) can be drawn: A person comes into being from the ground of *consciousness* and loses freedom as one is bound in *time* and finds one's identity in *space*. Matters of time-space are very much involved in one's struggles for self-determination and status. *Movement* represents the choice point. It is central to understanding the nature of reality. Through movement

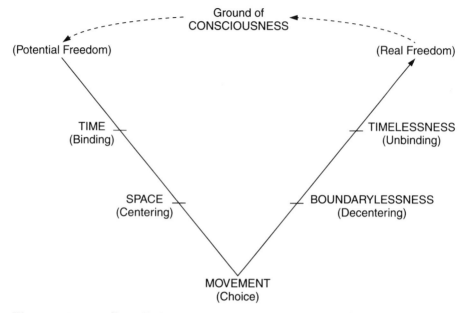

Figure 11.1   Parallel between Newman's Theory of Expanding Consciousness and Young's Stages of Human Evolution.

one discovers the world of time-space and establishes personal territory. It is also when movement is restricted that one becomes aware of personal limitations and the fact that the old rules don't work anymore. When one no longer has the power of movement (either physical or social), it is necessary to go beyond oneself. As one is able to recognize the *boundarylessness* and *timelessness* of human existence, one gains the freedom of returning to the ground of *consciousness*.

The transformation that occurs at the turning point may be understood from the stand-point of Prigogine's theory of change (Prigogine, Allen, & Herman, 1977). Prigogine asserts that the usual fluctuations of deterministic processes interact with chance events to bring about a kind of giant fluctuation that propels the system to another, higher level of organization and functioning. Disorder places a strain on the existing structure and is resisted by the structure. If the force of the fluctuation is great enough, the structure is forced to change and moves through a temporarily chaotic situation to a new higher order. Transformation takes place as the system moves far from equilibrium. The action at the critical point of the fluctuation has the potential to go in a number of directions, and it is impossible to know which way it will go. But at some point one direction takes over and a new order is established. In this new order, new rules apply.

The task at the choice point is discovering the new rules. It involves letting go of the control believed to exist in the binding/centering stages—the control, for instance, that some people think they have over health. Transcending one level of organization may mean going beyond the disease state, but there is no guarantee that this will occur. The task of transformation may mean moving into the freedom of infinite space-time in the presence of disease.

This unified concept of health includes disease as a meaningful manifestation of the underlying pattern and precludes a dichotomous view of health and disease. This perspective represents a paradigm shift. It requires letting go of the old, manipulative view of health in which one can *promote* health by adopting certain behaviors, *prevent* disease by avoiding other behaviors, and *cure* disease by submitting to prescribed treatments. This concept of health does not negate knowledge of disease and its treatment; it places such knowledge within the context of the whole rather than as the central focus.

Hence the paradigm that guides the theory of health as expanding consciousness is a paradigm of *evolving pattern of the whole*. The assumption is made that whatever manifests itself in a person's life is an explication of the underlying pattern. Disease, if it is present, is not a separate entity; it is a manifestation of the person's pattern of consciousness. Eliminating disease (the directive of the medical model) does not necessarily enhance the evolving pattern; actions toward this end may even dampen the pattern. What is needed is recognition of the pattern and its action potential.

Pattern recognition is key to the process of evolving to higher levels of consciousness. It occurs instantaneously and is "recognition of a principle, realization of a truth, reconciliation of a duality, *satori*" (Young, 1976, p. 180). It has been equated with insight and intuition. When it occurs, it illuminates the possibilities for action. It is like the difference between being in the dark and turning on the light; when the light comes on, one can see the possibilities for movement. Nursing facilitates this process by rhythmic connecting of the nurse with the client in an authentic way for the purpose of illuminating the pattern and discovering the new rules of a higher level of organization.

RESEARCH AS PRAXIS

There is a clarion call within the nursing profession for methodology consistent with the philosophical and theoretical perspective of the discipline. Early in the development of this concept of health, I realized that the phenomena of inquiry needed to be parameters of wholeness (Newman, 1979). Things such as the way a person moves or talks are enduring characteristics that identify a person across the life span. In this sense, the dimensions of person–environment interaction which form the framework for the current North American Nursing Diagnosis Association taxonomy (exchanging, communicating, relating, choosing, moving, feeling, valuing, perceiving, knowing) were helpful in forcing a holistic view of the interactive, dynamic nature of all of the phenomena at once (Newman, 1984). It was misleading, though, to try to fit all of the information gleaned about a person into one portrayal of the person's pattern. These phenomena are dynamic patterns of energy and are revealed in the nature of the flow of energy within the system and between the system and the environment. The pattern is unfolding over time—one configuration evolving into the next configuration, and so on. It is more helpful to portray the evolving pattern as sequential configurations over time (Newman, 1987a, 1987b). Such a portrayal is a step toward wholeness, but not enough. The nurse-researcher cannot stand outside the person being researched in a subject-object fashion. The researcher is part of the interaction pattern which is the process of pattern recognition and choice.

The elements of the research method currently being used to elaborate the pattern of expanding consciousness are: (a) establishing the mutuality of the process of inquiry, (b) focusing on the most meaningful persons and events in the interviewee's life, (c) organizing the data in narrative form and displaying it as sequential patterns over time, and (d) sharing the interviewer's perception of the pattern with the interviewee and seeking revision or confirmation (Newman, 1987b). Inherent in this process is the insight interviewees gain into their own pattern and the concomitant illumination of their action possibilities. This latter characteristic will be an essential purpose in future studies. The elements of this method are similar to the practice methodology described by Parse (1987, pp. 167–169), especially in relation to her emphasis on "illuminating meaning" and "mobilizing transcendence." Newman's method, however, embodies negotiation, reciprocity, and empowerment, characteristics of research as praxis.

The above method has been used in collaboration with people identified as experiencing various diseases (Jonsdottir, 1988; Moch, 1988; Newman, 1987b). Regardless of the level of the person's disease or disability, the action potential of their pattern of interaction focuses on their relationships with other people. The task they are facing—the rules they must discover—is how to engage in meaningful, reciprocal relationships. They want to talk about things that are important to them, to express a full range of emotions, and to be truly themselves. But often they do not know how. That is where nursing comes in.

Sometimes it is difficult to see the pattern as expanding consciousness in the present moment, but recognition of the action potential of the pattern will open the way for the transformation to occur. Even when the pattern appears to be disorganized or blocked, the direction of its unfolding is a higher level of consciousness.

SUMMARY

The theory of health as expanding consciousness is conceived within a paradigm of health and science emphasizing pattern of the evolving whole. It incorporates the self-organizing interplay of disorder and order, explicated as disease and absence of disease, in the process of moving to higher levels of consciousness. Some of the early research purported to test this theory stemmed form a mechanistic view of movement-space-time-consciousness and failed to honor the basic assumptions of the model. Current research focuses on the unfolding pattern of person-environment over time and incorporates the authentic involvement of the nurse researcher as a participant with the client in the process of expanding consciousness. This research exemplifies the interaction of theory and research as praxis.

REFERENCES

Bateson, G. (1979). *Mind and nature. A necessary unity.* New York: Dutton.

Bentov, I. (1978). *Stalking the wild pendulum.* New York: Dutton.

Bohm, D. (1980). *Wholeness and the implicate order.* London: Routledge & Kegan Paul.

Jonsdottir, H. (1988). *Health patterns of clients with chronic obstructive pulmonary disease.* Unpublished master's thesis, University of Minnesota, Minneapolis.

Lather, P. (1986). Research as praxis. *Harvard Educational Review, 56*(3), 257–277.

Moch, S. D. (1988). Health in illness: Experiences with breast cancer (Doctoral dissertation, University of Minnesota, 1988). *Dissertation Abstracts International, 50,* 47 b.

Morgan, G. (1983). Toward a more reflective social science. In G. Morgan (Ed.). *Beyond method: Strategies for social research* (pp. 368–376). Beverly Hills: Sage.

Newman, M. A. (1966). Identifying patient needs in short-span nurse-patient relationships. *Nursing Forum, 5*(1), 76–86.

Newman, M. A. (1972). Time estimation in relation to gait tempo. *Perceptual and Motor Skills, 34,* 359–366.

Newman, M. A. (1976). Movement tempo and the experience of time. *Nursing Research, 25,* 273–279.

Newman, M. A. (1979). *Theory development in nursing.* Philadelphia: F. A. Davis.

Newman, M. A. (1982). Time as an index of consciousness with age. *Nursing Research, 31,* 290–293.

Newman, M. A. (1983). Newman's health theory. In I. Clements & F. Roberts (Eds.), *Family health: A theoretical approach to nursing care* (pp. 161–175). New York: Wiley.

Newman, M. A. (1984). Nursing diagnosis: Looking at the whole. *American Journal of Nursing, 84,* 1496–1499.

Newman, M. A. (1986). *Health as expanding consciousness.* St. Louis: Mosby.

Newman, M. A. (1987a). Nursing's emerging paradigm: The diagnosis of pattern. In A. M. McLane (Ed.), *Classification of nursing* diagnoses: *Proceedings of the seventh conference, North American Nursing Diagnosis Association* (pp. 53–60). St. Louis: Mosby.

Newman, M. A. (1987b). Patterning. In M. Duffy & N. J. Pender (Eds.), *Conceptual issues in health promotion. Report of Proceedings of a Wingspread Conference* (pp. 36–50). Indianapolis: Sigma Theta Tau.

Newman, M. A., & Gaudiano, J. K. (1984). Depression as an explanation for decreased subjective time in the elderly, *Nursing Research, 33*(3), 137–139.

Newman, M. A., Vail, J. D., & Cowling. W. R. (1985). Unpublished pilot study.

Parse, R. R. (1987). *Nursing science: Major paradigms, theories and critiques.* Philadelphia: Saunders.

Prigogine, I., Allen, P. M., & Herman, R. (1977). In E. Laszlo & J. Bierman (Eds.), *Long-term trends in the evolution of complexity. Goals in a global community: The original background papers for Goals for Mankind* (Vol. 1) (pp 1–63). New York: Pergamon.

Reinharz, S. (1983). Phenomenology as a dynamic process. *Phenomenology and Pedagogy,* 1(1). 77–79.

Rogers, M. E. (1970). *An introduction to the theoretical basis of nursing.* Philadelphia: F. A. Davis.

Young, A. E. (1976). *The reflexive universe: Evolution of consciousness.* San Francisco: Robert Briggs.

CHAPTER TWELVE

Life Patterns of Persons with Coronary Heart Disease

Margaret A. Newman

Susan Diemert Moch

> *If a man has a seesaw in his voice, it will run into his sentences, into his poem, into the structure of his fable, into his speculation, into his charity.*
>
> Ralph Waldo Emerson

A CRITICAL DIMENSION of the theory of health as expanding consciousness is the assumption that disease, when present, is a manifestation of the evolving pattern of the whole (Newman, 1979, 1986, 1990). This assumption is supported by Bohm's theory of wholeness and the implicate order (Bohm, 1980). Bohm contends that the pattern which is manifest (in this case, the disease pattern) is an explication of the underlying implicate pattern of the whole. Likewise, from another perspective, there is evidence from fractal theory that gross patterns repeat themselves in greater and greater detail of pattern at sub-microscopic levels (Briggs & Peat, 1989). The position taken in this study is that the pattern of disease is a gross manifestation of an

Reprinted with permission from *Nursing Science Quarterly*, 4(4): 161–167, 1991.

underlying pattern that can be seen in behavioral patterns and in the pattern of inner experience of the person.

The pattern varies according to the unique configuration of each person-environment situation; however, the similarity of the disease pattern suggests that there will be similarity of patterns among persons with similar medical diagnoses. The objectives of this study were to describe the individual patterns of interaction of persons with coronary heart disease (CHD), to discern similarities and differences among the individual patterns, and to interpret these findings in terms of the conceptual congruence of the overall pattern with the theory of health as expanding consciousness.

Pattern identification is central to the theory and its application. Practicing nurses seek to recognize the individual, evolving pattern of the client in order to facilitate the client's insight and synchronization with the pattern. The significance of the study is twofold: (a) to illuminate the evolving patterns of this group of participants, and (b) to serve as a process guide for practicing nurses.

PROCEDURES

In selection of the sample, the medical diagnosis of CHD was chosen because of its prominence as a major health problem. A convenience sample of eleven persons (7 men and 4 women) who were clients in a cardiac rehabilitation program were interviewed while involved in the program. They were invited to participate in the study by a cardiovascular nursing specialist on the basis of her evaluation of their ability and readiness to be interviewed. Age and gender were not factors in the selection process; however, comparison of these factors indicated that the sample was reasonably representative of the clinic population. The mean age of the sample was 56 with women comprising 36% of the sample. The mean age of the women was 67, compared to 49 for the men. The mean age of the clinic population was 59 with women comprising 37% of the total; women's ages generally were approximately ten years older than the men.

Even though the investigators were aware, in general, of the literature regarding the personality types associated with heart disease, this study was undertaken in phenomenological fashion without specific attention to those types and with the intent of exploring in an open-ended way the participants' patterns of interaction over time. Interviews were conducted by the second author in offices at the center. As a step toward implementing an action research approach in which researcher and practitioner collaborate in carrying out the research, the cardiovascular nursing specialist in the rehabilitation center was considered a co-researcher and was co-interviewer as her schedule permitted. The nature and purpose of the interview as a collaboration between researchers and clients to understand the individual's overall life pattern was explained. Clients who were willing to participate signed a consent form in which the nature of the study and participants' rights to withdraw were described. All names used in this report are fictitious.

The interview began by asking the client to describe the most meaningful persons and events in her or his life. If prompting was needed, the participants were encouraged to think back over their lives and try to identify the persons or events that were most meaningful to them (Bramwell, 1984). The interviewers focused on what was meaningful to the client and followed the direction of the client in elaborating these experiences. The interviews were audiotaped, and after the initial interview, the tapes were reviewed and the data were organized into a chronological sequence of events and portrayed in a diagram of interpersonal relationships at critical points in their lives. (See Newman, 1987, portions of which appear in Chapters 7 and 8 of this book.) The nature of the evolving pattern was contemplated and discussed by the authors prior to a second interview, during which the interviewer shared the joint perception of the pattern with the interviewee and so-licited feedback regarding its accuracy and relevance. The recorded pattern was revised as indicated by the feedback from the participant.

A second, more intensive analysis of the transcripts of the interviews was conducted to articulate the pattern of the individual's relationships over time and to identify common themes in the evolving pattern of relationships. This analysis involved: (a) identifying the most important interactions and feelings described by the participant, (b) characterizing these highlights as themes of the individual pattern, (c) identifying themes common across several participants' patterns, and (d) identifying differences in the individual patterns. This process was repeated on a minimum of three occasions separated by one to two-month intervals.

FINDINGS

Similarities of Patterns

Three main themes surfaced as similar among the participants: (a) the need to excel, (b) the need to please others, and (c) the feeling of being alone.

The need to excel A predominant theme which emerged was the participants' need to excel: to be "*the best*," "*first*," "*No. 1.*" The satisfaction of being better than others and of winning was important to their sense of well-being. The *drive for perfection* was accompanied by their pleasure in being recognized for their accomplishments and in being the center of activity and in control. Here are some of their comments:

". . . anything I do . . . I do it right. . . . I'm somewhat of a perfectionist . . . I never took a back seat to anybody."

"I always like to win in sports . . . I didn't want to be just good, but better than whoever I competed with."

". . . one of the biggest highlights in life was I was the No. 1 mechanic in the shop. . . . the highlight of my life was I made my goal. . . . I felt like I had really made a mark in life."

"I loved [playing hockey] . . . the contact, . . . and getting out there and accomplishing, showing them you could do it. Hearing the fans, you know, your friends, rooting them on. That was great. I loved that. It's good for the ego."

"If you want something done right, you've got to do it yourself."

The need to please others   There was a strong need to please others and difficulty in expressing one's own feelings, especially in situations of conflict:

"I like to have other people satisfied with me and who I am. I like to satisfy other people."

"I had already done things that I didn't want to do [to please his wife] . . . I had made a lot of compromises . . . . I get very uncomfortable when I am in the middle of an argument."

"I always feel kind of obligated to help wherever help is needed."

". . . I never really talked to my girlfriend about anything like this [fear of dying in surgery]. We never really discuss anything, anything real important . . . you know, like life and death sort of thing."

"I never followed through with [hockey]. I was asked to leave the team because I was smoking, got me mad, ego trip, and I never went back out again, to play hockey for a team, but I should have."

"I'm a peaceful person, basically . . . sensitive. It's just I don't show it a lot . . . I just don't want enemies or hurt feelings between me and other friends people . . . . I'm a people pleaser."

The feeling of being alone   An even more pervasive theme was the feeling of being alone and a lack of connectedness to others. Several participants specifically described themselves as "loners." They described remembrance of an isolated childhood often within a family characterized by conflict, deprivation, alcoholism, or verbal abusiveness. They often experienced painful, seemingly loveless childhoods and they described experiences of being isolated and disconnected from their parents, siblings, and schoolmates. As adults they had conflictive or merely instrumental relationships with their spouses and children. They were usually more connected to their work or other community activities than to their families. A pattern of repeated episodes of disconnectedness could be seen in both their personal and work relationships over time, with alcoholism a common accompaniment to their difficulties. (See Table 12.1.)

Theoretically the similarities of pattern should reflect the pattern of the disease. Early research regarding behavioral patterns of persons with CHD portrayed them as being involved aggressively in "an incessant struggle to achieve more and more in less and less time," labeled as Type A (Friedman & Rosenman, 1974). They were thought to be motivated to assert and maintain control over their environment in order to avoid the fear of failure, and they were thought to have more stressful work experiences and marital relationships than their non-CHD counterparts. Further examination of the behavior of the coronary-prone person revealed the propensity to display hostility in explosive vocal mannerisms, and this characteristic was thought to be a discriminating factor (Dimsdale, 1988; Matthews, Glass, Rosenman, & Bortner, 1977). Dembroski and Costa (1988) delineated the type of hostility associated with CHD as antagonistic hostility, as seen in cynical, manipulative, and antagonistic attitudes and behavior.

Friedman and his associates, continuing to investigate the personality patterns associated with CHD have indicated that it is not simply a matter of the characteristics of the Type A, hard-driving, fast-moving, job-involved persons, versus Type B (the opposite of Type A) but that persons with CHD in *both* categories were *more repressed, more tense, illness-prone, and externally controlled*. Within the Type B category, the

Table 12.1 Participants' Descriptions of Aloneness, Lack of Connectedness

Allen*: Was the youngest in a large family and was designated the "last" to eat, so was afraid he would not get enough food. He described dissension with his siblings both as a child growing up and as an adult. His work was the most important thing in his life. His first wife left him because of the priority his work held in his life. He remarried. Began drinking heavily after first heart attack.

Bob: Said that he had no strong connections to anyone during childhood and adolescence. His parents fought frequently and divorced when he was age 13. He married at age 25 but always connected more to his work than to people. He drifted from his wife and began drinking heavily.

Carl: Referred to himself as always a loner, never interested in being with a gang: "I don't miss the crowd." He was one of nine children—a family in which it was emphasized that he was on his own.

Darlene: Her parents died when she was quite young, at which time she was separated from her siblings and sent to live with her aunt and uncle. She said that she had been lonely all her life.

David: Felt alone in performing chores around the house (sister and brother did not help). Said that he wished he could establish closeness in his own family (wife and two sons) but in talking about his wife's job, he expressed his wish not to participate in any way in her work. There was conflict with and distancing from his sons.

Ed: Said that his family was not close during childhood; he was scared of his abusive father and didn't have much respect for his mother. "The whole family was alcoholic." He has relied heavily on alcohol his entire life.

Frank: Talked about a painful, loveless childhood. Both parents were alcoholics. He said his father was a loner, "just like me." He felt pressured by his wife and had a tendency to "roam" to get away from the pressure and to seek solace in alcohol. He was separated from his wife and family for three years. His world was the bottle—he had no God, no relationship to anyone. But then he went back to his wife: "no place else to go."

Gary: Described himself as a loner. Felt disconnected from his family as a child and left home at age 15. After service in WWII he tried unsuccessfully to connect with father and siblings. He was married but saw it as a relationship of mutual exchange; he wanted meaningful connectedness with others but was unsure as to how to get it. He used alcohol to withdraw from others.

*All names are fictitious.

individuals with CHD may be motivated to be the center of attention but not have the social skills to accomplish their goal. They are seen as having poor coping behaviors and other traits that lead to frustration. They are characterized by "thwarted motives and high emotionality, which do not achieve suitable expressions" (Friedman, Hall, & Harris, 1985, p. 1313).

These latter findings are particularly consistent with the data of this study. The participants were not easily dichotomized in a Type A or Type B classification. Nearly all of them were motivated to excel, to be the center of attention and in control of their situations, but some often were thwarted in their ability to achieve success by their inability to assert themselves, their desire to please others, and often their escape into alcoholism.

The physical form that coronary heart disease takes may be envisioned grossly as a narrowing of the lumen of the arteries resulting from a buildup of the wall of the vessels, a situation which gradually decreases the blood supply (energy) to the heart. The functioning of the system may deteriorate gradually and may be disrupted precipitously by occlusion of the vessel. An analogous closing in on the life flow and expression of self in interpersonal relationships was illustrated in the interview data. The potential for opening up in a more expressive way was considered desireable. The crisis brought about by heart disease was viewed in different ways. One explanation stems from the participants' locations on the developmental spectrum.

Differences Among Individual Patterns

Young's spectrum of human development is integral to the theory of health as expanding consciousness and provides an explanation for the differences observed in individual patterns (Newman, 1986; 1990; Young, 1978). Figure 12.1 depicts Young's (1978) sequencing of human evolution. The first stage of development, according to Young, is characterized by *binding,* a phase in which everything is

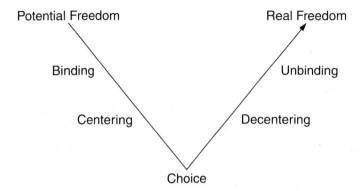

Figure 12.1   Young's Sequencing of Human Evolution.

regulated for the individual who is sacrificed for the sake of the collective. There is very little individual identity or choice here.

The second stage, *centering,* is one in which the individual seeks to establish her or his identity by striving for success in the material and power sense. The stage is characterized by self-determination, competitiveness, and seeking control over others.

The next stage in Young's spectrum, *choice,* comes about when something happens that forces the individual to recognize that these self-determined strivings do not work anymore, that they are not really bringing about the "progress" they were seeking. It is a time of choice, a turning point at which the task of the individual is to discover how things work in this new reality and to move beyond the old ways to a reality not limited by the space-time dimensions of the physical world. The crisis of a heart attack or coronary surgery may represent such an event. This stage is central as an explanatory theory for practicing nurses as they encounter persons facing these choices. The transcendent phase of Young's spectrum begins when there is a shift from emphasis on self to concern with development beyond self.

The individual patterns seen in this study cluster around the binding, centering, and choice phases of Young's spectrum, differing by the extent to which participants were able to establish their identity. There were glimpses of a shift to the transcendent arm of the spectrum in the participants who experienced the coronary event as an opportunity to consider major life changes. Also, two older women whose individual patterns revealed well-integrated patterns seemed to have progressed beyond the self-centered characteristics of the binding and centering stages (Barbara and Darlene). Two other participants who died during the period of the study revealed the disorganization and turbulence that occurs in a system prior to transformation (See descriptions of Ann and Ed).

Binding Stage

There were several examples of individual patterns depicting the binding stage. Carol, Frank, and David felt they had missed their opportunity to pursue a meaningful career and seemed to be still searching for who they were and how to relate to others. They felt controlled by others, and Carol particularly felt as though she had sacrificed her life for the sake of her family. They recognized their physical condition as a reminder of their mortality and limited life span, and they were unable to see beyond the bind they were in:

CAROL (age 59) saw herself as limited by her obligations to her family, both when she was a child and presently as a mother and wife. She felt she had "missed the boat" regarding the development of a career and never accomplished anything for herself. She felt she was expected to be available to her family. She regarded her capabilities as limited: that she was inadequate as wife and mother and a failure because two of her children had turned away from her teachings. She saw herself as going round in circles, like "a squirrel in a cage."

FRANK (age 41) referred to himself as a "people pleaser." When he "started moving along and getting involved" (in AA), he was sober and happy, but then his wife thought he was putting too much into it, and he started easing up, skipping meetings, and started drinking again: "I let her get to me."

For DAVID (age 44), his experience as a hockey player in high school was the highlight of his life. He revelled in his ability to win, to show what he could do. All of that came to a halt when he was kicked off the team for smoking. He got mad and sulked away without ever trying to get back on the team. In the interview David expressed regret that he "never followed through with [the hockey]" ". . . That's probably what I should have done right from the beginning . . . stay with it . . . and get on with what you want to do." David felt that his life pretty much stopped following coronary artery bypass surgery. His inactivity was depressing to him, made even more so by the realization that he may not have much time left.

Centering Stage

The experiences of Allen and Carl represent examples of individual patterns depicting the centering stage. Allen and Carl were able to accomplish what they had set out to do in their careers, but then experienced the disruption and loss of this ability due to physical limitations related to heart disease.

The most important thing to ALLEN (age 57) was that he be intensely involved in things and get them done "right." He has worked hard all his life to satisfy other people and to be highly regarded in the community. He has worked his way up to being the head of the family business. He said he "didn't take a back seat to anybody." In addition, he became the administrator of the volunteer fire department. This work was the "biggest part" of his life. He prided himself in being the first person on the scene for twenty years.

He expressed pride and satisfaction in being in the center and at the helm of helping activities, and although he had to cut down on his work activities after his acute episode of coronary heart disease, he was still enjoying first place as a "supergrandpa" to his grandson.

CARL (age 46) did not know what to do next. His entire life had been devoted to following his mother's admonitions to find the "right" job and become the best at what he did. He went through a great many jobs before becoming an auto mechanic and working up to be the No. 1 mechanic. Carl also became very involved in lodge activities and became the "No. 1" man and was "known all over [the state]." He enjoyed the sense of being in charge and seeing the whole picture. He was pleased with his role in helping and advising others and found his relationship to his lodge brothers very meaningful.

Choice Stage

Some participants were able to move beyond their current situation and view the heart attack or the bypass surgery as a critical time of re-evaluation of the meaning and direction of their lives. Bob, for example, epitomized someone who had experienced all of the same strivings for the top position and for perfection as did Allen and Carl. But, Bob was moving on and clearly experiencing the disruption in his life brought on by the heart attack as a *turning point,* a choice point, from which he could move beyond the space-time limitations of his past into a higher dimension of being.

As a boy BOB (age 38) developed skills in both music and sports and enjoyed excelling in what he did. He liked the competition and liked to win, to be better than everyone else. He said he was never closely connected to anyone but did marry at the age of 25. His love for and commitment to his music as a career took precedence over his marriage. For a while he had made decisions regarding his work to please his wife, but later was unwilling to compromise what he wanted to do, and they divorced. Bob played with a series of bands, going from one to the other, thinking he would find the perfect one but eventually they all ended up in bickering and would break up. He began drinking heavily after his separation from his wife as part of the lifestyle of his work.

Bob's heart attack was like a *"turning point"* for him. He had been questioning what the message was in this, what the reasons were for things happening. He felt like he was becoming more spiritual:

"I do believe that there is a higher power. I am open to all kinds of different concepts. Maybe it's time for a change . . . Maybe this is something I should take advantage of, maybe there is something I can contribute. I just don't know where to begin."

"I think of things because I have had a heart attack that . . . I would never be thinking . . . I'd be having the time of my life right now probably . . . I'm thinking of possibly doing something else than what I am doing up to this point, and you know, if I hadn't had the heart attack, I wouldn't be considering anything else . . . This could be the best thing that ever happened to [me]."

GARY (age 60), too, had already been experiencing the need to "remodel" his life at the time of his heart attack and showed signs of transcending his previous limitations. He was in the process of remodeling his home when he had a heart attack. He had quit drinking and was getting ready to retire when it occurred. He expressed a sense of "wanting more" from his relationships with his family and the possibility that "maybe [he just hasn't] grown up yet." He was seeking a closer relationship with his family and related greater affectionate expressiveness.

Transcendent Stage

BARBARA and DARLENE were both considerably older than the other participants (70s compared to primarily 40s and 50s). They expressed some of the characteristics already described, but were more connected with their families and community than the other participants and seemed to have less need for control. They presented a more fully integrated pattern that probably falls somewhere on the transcendent arm of Young's spectrum. Their heart attacks, viewed from the vantage point of long lives of complex relationships and events, did not seem to represent the same degree of disruption as it did for the others.

The greater integration of the patterns of these two women's lives may relate to their age and socialization as women. Bateson (1989) has described the ability of women, by virtue of their responsibilities to husband and children, to integrate interruptions in their personal and career development.

Disorganization and Death

Two participants died during the conduct of the study. The first was a woman 56 years old. Prior to her heart attack the most important thing in ANN'S life had been being able to take care of her own affairs, run her home, maintain order, and keep things running smoothly. But she was no longer able to do that. For the past six months she had been unable to run her home and deal with her affairs. She felt disconnected, disordered. She was afraid of everything, had lost her confidence in her ability to do anything. She felt as though her "world has collapsed right on top of [her]." The evening after Ann was interviewed, she collapsed and died at home.

ED, 59 years old, had been experiencing fatigue, depression, and no motivation to go on following his heart attack. In the days prior to his death, he had decided not to undergo further treatment but was unable to follow through with that decision. He reported several days of irritability and nights of insomnia, and expressed disgust at becoming a cardiac cripple. Ed's personal distress was intense; he wanted to go home or take a vacation. He didn't care about the consequences. With recurrent chest pain, however, he did not leave the hospital. Instead he underwent bypass surgery, during which he died.

The place of disorder in the self-organizing capacity of the living system is relevant (Prigogine, 1976). Turbulence, the point of shift from order to disorder, is a sign of the system's deep interconnectedness with the whole and is a critical point in a person's transformation (Briggs & Peat, 1989). Both of the above participants evidenced turbulence in their lives prior to their deaths.

PATTERN CONCLUSIONS

The theory of health as expanding consciousness incorporates positions regarding pattern that appear paradoxical. The theory is based on the assumption of pattern as identifying the unique, evolving wholeness of the person. At the same time the theory embraces disease as a manifestation of the pattern of the person. These statements imply that each individual is characterized by a unique configuration of person-environment interaction over time, and that individuals who have the same disease manifest the same pattern. It is this paradox that this study intended to address. The findings support both sides of the paradox: The individual patterns were unique to each individual's situation, and there were patterns of interaction that were similar among the participants of the study. The similar patterns represent developmental tasks related to the first rung of Young's (1978) theory of human evolution. When those developmental needs were frustrated or when individuals were caught in a repetitive cycle of self-aggrandizement characteristic of the centering stage, the blocks to movement along the spectrum experienced by the participants were mirrored in the blocks in the disease process. The individual differences were apparent as some participants moved further along in the spectrum of development, and the differences were accentuated when participants faced the critical choice point that the manifestation of the disease represented. If they reached the choice point early enough and still had enough resources to confront their pattern and allow the meaning of their pattern to unfold, they had the potential of transcending the physical limitations and moving beyond themselves to a higher level of consciousness. If they had reached the limits of their resources, death was "the transformative door" (Moss, 1981, p. 101) to higher consciousness. One might speculate that if participants had experienced this process of pattern identification prior to the manifestation of the disease, they could have gotten in "sync" with their patterns before it became necessary for the pattern to emerge in the form of disease.

IMPLICATIONS FOR PRACTICE

According to J. Huebsch, the cardiovascular nursing specialist involved in this study, this process of pattern identification can be easily incorporated into clinicians' daily activities with clients. Huebsch points out that the interviews "added enormously to the information base of each patient even when I thought I knew the patients." The process can be engaged in by the nurse to open up the experience of the clients and to connect authentically as person to person to the clients' situations. Huebsch emphasizes the importance of clinicians experiencing the process and recommends that for future research the schedule be set up to incorporate a staff member in each interview.

Huebsch examined the pattern conclusions of this study in light of her personal knowledge of the participants, and agreed that the patterns described fit the data but cannot be construed to fit all coronary heart disease patients. Most of the research on interpersonal patterns in relation to CHD does seek to generalize to the entire population and is aimed at detection of persons at risk for CHD for the purpose of preventing the disease. In addition, there are certain lifestyle changes related to diet, exercise, smoking, and stress management that are considered important in the prevention of, and rehabilitation from, the disease (Frenn, Borgeson, Lee, & Simandl, 1989).

This study offers a different perspective, one that emphasizes the meaning of the disruption that CHD represents for each person. The emphasis is on the unfolding pattern of the individual person's life and the importance of helping the individual get in touch with her or his pattern and express herself or himself more fully. The things that were most meaningful to the participants of this study were: (a) a sense of who they were, (b) a need to develop better relationships with members of their family, and (c) a desire to discover a new way of life. But often they did not know how to go about pursuing these objectives.

That's where nursing practice comes in. The presence of another person who is sensitive to self and to the environment can facilitate accomplishment of these objectives by mirroring the client's pattern. Participating in the client's pattern recognition, and what it represents in terms of the individual's stage of human development, opens the way to movement along the evolutionary spectrum.

The practice implications of this study relate more to the process than to the content. The process enacted through this research occurs as a nurse and client come together and form a shared consciousness (Newman, 1986, 1989). This rhythmic process of coming together and moving apart occurs until the client is able to see clearly and take action to express her or his "truth."

REFERENCES

Bateson, M. C. (1989). *Composing a life*. New York: The Atlantic Monthly Press.

Bohm, D. (1980). *Wholeness and the implicate order*. London: Routledge & Kegan Paul.

Bramwell, L. (1984). Use of the life history in pattern identification and health promotion. *Advances in Nursing Science, 7*, 37–44.

Briggs, J., & Peat, F. D. (1989). *Turbulent mirror*. New York: Harper & Row.

Dembroski, T. M., & Costa, P. T. (1988). Assessment of coronary-prone behavior: A current overview. *Annals of Behavioral Medicine, 10,* 60–63.

Dimsdale, J. E. (1988). A perspective on type A behavior and coronary disease. *The New England Journal of Medicine, 318,* 110–112.

Frenn, M. D., Borgeson, D. S., Lee, H. A., & Simandl, G. (1989). Lifestyle changes in a cardiac rehabilitation program: The client perspective. *Journal of Cardiovascular Nursing, 3,* 43–55.

Friedman, H. S., Hall, J. A., & Harris, M. J. (1985). Type A behavior, nonverbal expressive style, and health. *Journal of Personality and Social Psychology, 48,* 1299–1315.

Friedman, M., & Rosenman, R. H. (1974). *Type A behavior and your heart.* New York: Knopf.

Matthews, K. A., Glass, D. C., Rosenman, R. H., & Bortner, R. W. (1977). Competitive drive, pattern A, and coronary heart disease: A further analysis of some data from the western collaborative group study. *Journal of Chronic Disease, 30,* 489–498.

Moss, R. (1981). *The I that is we.* Millbrae, CA: Celestial Arts.

Newman, M. A. (1979). *Theory development in nursing.* Philadelphia: Davis.

Newman, M. A. (1986). *Health as expanding consciousness.* St. Louis: Mosby.

Newman, M. A. (1987). Patterning. In M. Duffy & N. J. Pender (Eds.), *Conceptual issues in health promotion.* A report of proceedings of a Wingspread conference. Indianapolis: Sigma Theta Tau.

Newman, M. A. (1989). The spirit of nursing. *Holistic Nursing Practice, 3*(3), 1–6.

Newman, M. A. (1990). Newman's theory of health as praxis. *Nursing Science Quarterly, 3,* 37–41.

Prigogine, I. (1976). Order through fluctuation: Self-organization and social system. In E. Jantsch & C. H. Waddington (Eds.), *Evolution and consciousness.* (pp. 93–133.) Reading, Mass.: Addison-Wesley.

Young, A. M. (1978). *The reflexive universe: Evolution of consciousness.* San Francisco: Robert Briggs.

CHAPTER THIRTEEN

Recognizing a Pattern of Expanding Consciousness in Persons with Cancer

Margaret A. Newman

THE PURPOSE OF this study is to continue to examine the theory of health as expanding consciousness from the standpoint of the life pattern of persons manifesting major disease configurations. An assumption of this theory is that disease, when present, is a manifestation of the evolving pattern of the whole and can provide insight into the human needs of the person who is engaged in the developmental process of expanding consciousness (Newman, 1986). The objective of this particular study was to explore the meaning of the life pattern of several persons diagnosed with cancer in terms of their interaction with the environment, and to identify differences in relation to their position on Young's spectrum of human development (Young, 1978). The findings were examined from the perspective of the theory of health as expanding consciousness and the implications for nursing practice.

BACKGROUND OF THE THEORY

The idea of disease as a manifestation of a primary, underlying pattern of the person was stimulated by the theory of complementarity set forth by Bahnson and Bahnson (1966) in the early sixties. These investigators hypothesized that humans have two basic ways to discharge the energy continuously generated in their person–environment interaction: one is to discharge it in their actions on the external environment, the other is to direct it internally in somatic changes. Accordingly, the diseases that these two types of individuals manifest would take the form of the underlying universal pattern, e.g., schizophrenia in the instance of external behavioral manifestations, and cancer in internal manifestations.

This theoretical position is consistent with the assumption of pattern as the identifying factor of one's unique wholeness (Rogers, 1970) and with the assumption that disease is a manifestation of the pattern of the whole (Newman, 1979, 1986).

Further, these assumptions are supported by physicist David Bohm's (1980) theory of wholeness and the implicate order. The implicate order is an unseen, underlying pattern that is primary and manifests itself from time to time in an explicate pattern, a physical reality that is observable through our senses. The explicate order is a manifestation of the implicate order and moves in and out of our manifest reality. (One way to visualize this phenomenon is to think of the ocean as the implicate order and the waves as the explicate order, making their appearance from time to time in observable form and then going back into the vastness of the ocean.) Within the context of the theory of health as expanding consciousness, disease is viewed as the explication of the underlying pattern of the wholeness of the person in interaction with the environment.

The premise that persons with similar diseases have similar interactive patterns is incomplete without consideration of the uniqueness of the pattern of each person–environment trajectory across space-time. In a study combining these points of view there should be similarities of the overall interactive pattern for persons having the same disease and differences in pattern related to each person's particular position in space-time.

Based on these premises, a previous study on life patterns of persons with coronary heart disease (Newman & Moch, 1991) was undertaken. The data revealed patterns that were similar to those found in the literature on personality types associated with heart disease, but also differences associated with points on the spectrum of human development proposed by Young (1978).

Young includes five stages of development: binding, centering, choice, decentering and unbinding. In the first stage, binding, the individual is sacrificed for the sake of the collective. Everything is regulated for the individual, for whom there is very little individual identity or choice. In the second stage, centering, individuals seek to establish their identities via success in the material and power sense. Self-determination, competitiveness, and seeking control over others are characteristics of this stage. The next stage, choice, comes about when the individual realizes that these self-centered strivings "do not work" anymore. It is a time of choice, a turning point, at which the individual seeks to discover how to move beyond the old ways to a reality not limited by the space-time dimensions of the physical world. The transcendent phase of Young's spectrum, the decentering and unbinding stages, comes about as a person shifts from emphasis on self to concern with development beyond the self.

For example, the aggressive, competitive behaviors commonly associated with heart patients seeking to be at the top of their field were apparent in a number of participants, but some had accomplished this goal, which might be classified as having achieved the centering stage of Young's spectrum, and were at a turning point of choosing (choice stage) to move to more spiritual kinds of experiences (transcendent stages). Whereas others were still caught in repetitive actions (between binding and centering), trying to find out who they were and how to relate to others.

Interpretive emphasis on the individuality of pattern is particularly relevant to nursing science since the practice of nursing focuses in part on the application of this research to individuals and their families. It pinpoints where the individual is in the overall scheme of expanding consciousness and suggests what the nurse might anticipate as the next stage of the evolving pattern of a client.

PROCEDURES

The participants for this study were four men and three women, all of whom had been diagnosed as having cancer. They ranged in age from 35 to 80 years old. They were patients in an outpatient clinic in a large, metropolitan health center which serves a generally middle-class population. They were invited to participate in the study by a cancer nursing specialist from patients receiving follow-up care at the time of the study. There were no exclusionary criteria such as site, type or stage of the disease. The intent of the study was to examine the life pattern of the participants in relation to the theory of health as expanding consciousness; there was no intent to generalize regarding risk factors related to cancer.

The nature and purpose of the study was explained to prospective participants. They were told that the purpose of the study was to learn about life patterns as they relate to health. The procedure involved two taped interviews of approximately 45 minutes to one hour. Clients who were willing to participate signed a consent form in which the nature of the study and participants' rights to withdraw were described. Interviews were conducted in a private room near the clinic by a master's prepared nurse who was knowledgeable about the Newman theory and was skilled in non-directive interviewing. The cancer nursing specialist also participated in the interviews as her schedule permitted. All names used in this report are pseudonyms.

The procedures for data collection and analysis were identical to those used in a previous study of persons with coronary heart disease (Newman & Moch, 1991). The interview began by establishing the mutuality of the nurse-interviewer and client in a cooperative endeavor to identify the meaning in the client's life pattern. The client was asked to describe the most meaningful persons and events in her or his life. If prompting was needed, the participants were encouraged to think back over their lives to try to identify the persons or events that were most meaningful to them. The interviewer focused on what was meaningful to the clients and followed the direction of the client in elaborating these experiences. The interviews were audiotaped.

After the initial interview, the tape was reviewed and the data were organized into a chronological sequence of events and portrayed in a diagram of interpersonal relationships at critical points in their lives (Newman, 1987). There was no interpretation of data at this point; the emerging individual pattern of interrelationships was shared with the interviewee, who was asked for feedback regarding its accuracy and relevance. The derived pattern was revised as indicated by the feedback from the participant.

A second, more intensive analysis of the transcripts of the interviews was conducted to identify themes in the evolving pattern of relationships. This analysis involved: (a) identifying what appeared to be the most important interactions and feelings described by the participant, (b) characterizing these highlights as themes of the individual pattern, (c) identifying themes common across several participants' patterns, and (d) identifying differences in the individual patterns. The individual patterns were then compared with the Young spectrum of evolving consciousness (Newman, 1990).

This hermeneutic, dialectic method of inquiry establishes the participants as co-investigators in the search for the most meaningful times in their lives. The interviewer's ability to be fully present in the interview and to follow the lead of the interviewee in telling his or her story is an important factor in maintaining the credibility of the narrative. Verification of the accuracy of the pattern was ascertained in the second interview during which the interviewer offers back to the interviewee a chronological, diagrammed pattern. Subsequent interpretation of the data is based on the author's understanding of the theory. Readers can judge for themselves whether or not the data presented is consistent with the proposed themes and definitions. The selection of data in relation to this particular theoretical perspective does not preclude support for other theories. The findings are not meant to be predictive. They provide retrospective illumination of the participants' patterns, and guidance for the process of nursing practice in facilitating clients' insight regarding their evolving patterns.

SIMILARITY OF PATTERNS

Deprived Childhood

The most predominant theme that emerged from the interview data was the experience of a deprived, difficult childhood and a kind of weariness or rejection of their lives, from a retrospective view. The deprivation was manifested in poverty, disease, separation from significant others, abusive parents, or a combination of these factors. The following sketches illustrate the participants' recalled experiences of poverty, illness and abuse:

> **Adam*** talked about growing up in a very poor family and going to work when he was 8 or 9 years old: "I didn't get a chance to play as much athletics as I wanted to. I worked every day in the week in the summer time. I'd leave home at 3:30 in the morning, and I'd get home about 7:00 at night . . . we either worked or starved."

> **Bryan** had pneumonia as a child and did not walk until he was 3 years old. He felt close to his mother but was rejected by his father and "yearned for a normal home."

> **Charles** described a childhood of "hard times." He went to work early to help his family.

* All names of participants used in this report are pseudonyms.

Dana had severe infectious diseases as a child. At the age of 14 she had tuberculosis and was sent to a sanitorium for 7 months. This meant she had to drop out of school and eventually was 2 years behind her original class. She was unable to participate in sports.

Frances' mother died when she was 2 years old, and she became an orphan. "All I can remember is working." She was kicked out of the orphanage when she was 10 years old. At that time she became a housekeeper for her father and brother, but "things went badly." She was then placed in a foster home, where she worked for her room and board. She said there was never any time for school. She became a ward of the state at age 15 and was released at age 20.

George was punished harshly as a child by his father. His mother was supportive to the children but submissive to his father.

This theme is consistent with the findings of Kune and his associates that cancer patients reported childhood or adult life 'unhappiness' (Kune, Kune, Watson, & Bahnson, 1991). Only one participant in this study referred to her childhood situation in a positive way, but even in this situation, the emphasis was on the basic necessities of life, such as food and clothing.

Lack of Connectedness

A related theme was the feeling of lack of connectedness with other people:

Adam said that his life had been "uneventful." Retired at the time of the interview, he said he was active in the community and had lots of friends but that he "had never really been really close to anybody."

Brian says he thinks a lot about suicide: "When I look at my life, it seems like it has been a series of failures . . . I just want to die a lot. . . . there is a lot of meaningless disconnectedness . . . I want companionship. I want connectedness."

Evelyn feels her life was "tragic" because her husband left her when her children were small. She is in a nursing home now and feels stripped of her possessions and her way of life. She feels alone.

The above comments are consistent with reports from other research portraying cancer patients as living unhappy, drab lives. Depression and hopelessness are part of a constellation of factors associated with the lives of persons who have cancer (Temoshok, 1987; Shekelle et al., 1981). The presence of cancer is correlated with a number of traumatic events evoking chronic hopelessness (Grossarth-Maticek & Eysenck, 1990).

TURNING POINTS

In spite of a long history of self-sacrifice and abrogation of their own needs in favor of others, some of the participants, having faced the diagnosis of cancer and other losses in their lives, reached a turning point at which they were able to transcend their limitations. Here are some examples:

Frances spent her life taking care of others, first as a child and later as a young adult. After just getting married, she went to another city to take care of her ill sister. Then her husband was killed shortly thereafter. Later she remarried, but her second husband was abusive. Even so she took care of him after he had had surgery. She is now in a nursing home where the staff is very warm and caring. Frances said, "I've never had any warmth in my life . . . All I ever had was rejection, but they [nursing home staff] were really helpful . . . they gave me back the will to live. For once I could show my warmth."

Dana's mother committed suicide when Dana was 19 years old; so she stayed home and took care of the family. Her younger brother, aged 6, was killed in an auto accident while she was taking care of him. She married at age 24 and had two children, but her husband was sick a lot (was hospitalized in the

State hospital), and she feels that she raised the children alone. By age 68, she had had 5 surgeries (for cataracts and several types of cancer) in 6 years. But she seems to have transcended these problems and is happy and at peace with her family: "I used to worry about the future, but now since I got the cancer, I live one day at a time . . . I am happy now."

Charles married early and divorced his wife when he found out she had been unfaithful to him. His second wife shared his interests and was responsible for reviving him from a near-death experience. She is still by his side through his experience [of two bouts of cancer, surgery, chemotherapy and physical therapy]. He appears to have transcended his physical problems and to be enjoying his life with family and friends.

George had been engaged to his wife for several years but did not get married until he was diagnosed with cancer. His wife is very caring and tends to "take care of" him. Since being diagnosed with cancer, he says "I don't take things for granted anymore. I appreciate every special thing that happens."

The pattern of interaction of nearly all of the participants in this study would fit the binding stage of Young's spectrum, a stage characterized by being bound by external demands and self-sacrifice. The crisis of their experience with cancer brought some to a turning point of living more fully what remains of their lives in the present. The experience of cancer did help some of them to move beyond their difficulties to a greater appreciation for their lives.

LeShan (1989) sees cancer as a turning point in people's lives in terms of finding "more experience of the self, self-recognition and the recognition—and often fulfillment—of dreams." Regardless of whether the person is in a living or dying mode, "the essence of the task . . . is to see the whole of our lives as a pattern and a symphony . . ." LeShan observes that the patients he has worked with are ready to explore the pattern of their lives. He emphasizes that ". . . our ultimate concern" [is] "the growth of our own being. Or, if you will, the development of our soul." Most people, he points out, "are capable of finding this out in the last days *if they have caring and concerned help.*" [Emphasis added]

HEALTH AS EXPANDING CONSCIOUSNESS

Moch's examination of the theory of health as expanding consciousness from the standpoint of the experience of women with breast cancer revealed a changing relatedness of these women with both their physical and interpersonal surroundings (Moch, 1990). They described ways in which they had become more sensitive to their own needs. They felt closer to others and were more receptive to others' expressions of caring. In general, they felt a greater connectedness and a greater appreciation of life. The enhanced quality of their interactions was seen as an indicator of the expansion of consciousness.

The assumption of the theory of health as expanding consciousness is that life is proceeding in the direction of higher consciousness. From this perspective, cancer can be experienced as a turning point, a choice point, at which persons become more fully themselves. Some, like those in this study, have been caught in the bind of living their lives for others, unable to experience the essence of their own being. In the crisis of cancer and the reality of their own mortality, they may be able to open up to more meaningful relationships (Reed, 1991). The transcendence of the limitations of the disease does not necessarily mean freedom from the disease (although in some cases this occurs); it does mean more meaningful relationships and greater freedom in a spiritual sense. The process of getting in touch with one's own pattern, being more authentic in one's relationships and transcending self limitations is a manifestation of expanding consciousness.

For those persons with cancer who do not show evidence of expanding consciousness, "death may be the transformative door" (Moss, 1981). Or, the absence of observable evidence may be a function of the observer; the ability to see pattern is in the eye of the beholder (Newman, 1983). Experience in studying and applying this theory indicates that the transforming power of the theory manifests itself as it is applied.

IMPLICATIONS FOR NURSING

Currently calls are being issued across many disciplines for greater emphasis on helping people find meaning in their lives (International Transpersonal Association, 1992). The nursing profession, with its commitment to caring, is in a prime position to assist persons to get in touch with their own patterns, the meaning of their lives. The nursing home experience of Frances (described on p. 166) of being cared for and of feeling her own warmth toward others brought a new sense of meaning and will to live. The nursing staff made it possible for this woman to experience the connectedness she had never experienced before.

The short-term implications of the findings of this study for nursing practice is the need people have for connectedness, relatedness. Key words the participants used to describe their lives were "uneventful," "tragic," "insecure," "abused," "lack of warmth," and "disconnected." A caring nurse, whether in the hospital, the clinic, the nursing home, or hospice facility, can be fully present and enter into the process of pattern identification with the client. Through that connectedness the individuals may find meaning in their pattern and may begin to experience their own caring and warmth, as did Frances.

The procedures used in this study to identify pattern can be used by the practicing nurse to facilitate this process. The necessary ingredients are: (1) being fully present, (2) seeking to know about the most meaningful experiences in the client's life, and (3) mirroring this story for the client so that they can see the evolving pattern. The nurse must be sensitive to thoughts and feelings that arise and recognize that they are manifestations of the field of interpenetration of both client and nurse.

The long-term implications of this study for health are the general needs for connectedness and nurturing. The increasing incidence of poverty and homelessness in our society suggests the prevalence of these needs. People should not have to wait until the manifestation of disease brings them to the attention of "caring and concerned help."

REFERENCES

Bahnson, C. B., & Bahnson, M. G. (1966). Role of the ego defenses: Denial and repression in the aetiology of malignant neoplasm. In C. B. Bahnson & D. M. Kissen (Eds.), Psychophysiological aspects of cancer. *Annals of the New York Academy of Science, 125,* 827–845.

Bohm, D. (1980). *Wholeness and the implicate order.* London: Routledge & Kegan Paul.

Grossarth-Maticek, R., & Eysenck, H. J. (1990). Coffee-drinking and personality as factors in the genesis of cancer and coronary heart disease. *Neuropsychobiology, 23,* 153–159.

International Transpersonal Association. (1992). Conference in Prague, Czechoslovakia, June, 1992.

Kune, G. A., Kune, S., Watson, L. F., & Bahnson, C. B. (1991). Personality as a risk factor in large bowel cancer: Data from the Melbourne colorectal cancer study. *Psychological Medicine, 21,* 29–41.

LeShan, L. (1989). Cancer as a turning point. *Noetic Sciences Review, 11,* 22–28.

Moch, S. D. (1990). Health within the experience of breast cancer. *Journal of Advanced Nursing, 15,* 1426–1435.

Moss, R. (1981). *The I that is we.* Millbrae, CA: Celestial Arts.

Newman, M. A. (1979). *Theory development in nursing.* Philadelphia: F. A. Davis.

Newman, M. A. (1983). Editorial. *Advances in Nursing Science, 5*(2), x–xi.

Newman, M. A. (1986). *Health as expanding consciousness.* St. Louis: C. V. Mosby.

Newman, M. A. (1987). Patterning. In M. Duffy & N. J. Pender (Eds.), *Conceptual issues in health promotion. Report of proceedings of a Wingspread Conference* (pp. 36–50). Indianapolis: Sigma Theta Tau.

Newman, M. A. (1990). Newman's theory of health as praxis. *Nursing Science Quarterly, 3,* 37–41.

Newman, M. A., & Moch, S. D. (1991). Life patterns of persons with coronary heart disease, *Nursing Science Quarterly, 4,* 161–167.

Reed, P. G. (1991). Toward a nursing theory of self-transcendence: Deductive reformulation using developmental theories. *Advances in Nursing Science, 13*(4), 64–77.

Rogers, M. E. (1970). *An introduction to the theoretical basis of nursing.* Philadelphia: F. A. Davis.

Shekelle, R. B., Raynor, W. F., Jr., Ostfeld, A. M., Garron, D. C., Bieliauskas, L. A., Liu, S. C., Maliza, C., & Oglesby, P. (1981). Psychological depression and 17-year risk of death from cancer. *Psychosomatic Medicine, 43*(2), 117–125.

Temoshok, L. (1987). Personality, coping style, emotion and cancer: Towards an integrative model. *Cancer Surveys, 6*(3), 545–567.

Young, A. M. (1978). *The reflexive universe: Evolution of consciousness.* San Francisco: Robert Briggs.

Author Notes

I would like to express my appreciation to Susan D. Moch, PhD, RN, and Shirley Williams, RN, for their assistance in the implementation of this study.

CHAPTER FOURTEEN

The Paradox of HIV/AIDS as Expanding Consciousness

Frank P. Lamendola

Margaret A. Newman

THE PHENOMENON OF the human immunodeficiency virus (HIV)/
acquired immunodeficiency syndrome (AIDS) has captured the concern and imagination of a full spectrum of life scientists. Nursing scientists have focused primarily on the caring, experiential aspects of
living and dying with HIV/AIDS and the associated anguish
and loss of the communities experiencing this phenomenon (Belcher,
Dettmore, & Holzemer, 1989; Carson, Soeken, Shanty, & Terry, 1990;
Carson & Green, 1992; Gloersen, et al., 1993; Hall, 1990; Korniewicz,
O'Brien, & Larson, 1990; Nokes & Carver, 1991; Ragsdale & Morrow, 1990; Sowell et al., 1991). The paradoxical nature of living and
dying faced by all human beings is personified in those who are HIV
positive or have AIDS. The nursing theory of health as expanding consciousness is particularly relevant, since the theory incorporates disease
as a manifestation of the evolving pattern of the whole person in
interaction with the environment (Newman, 1979, 1986, 1990).
Consciousness, the total information of the person (physiologic as well
as cognitive and affective), is manifested in the pattern of person-
environment interaction, including self-transcendent experiences.

The meaning of HIV/AIDS has been expanded by cultural historian William Irwin Thompson, systems theorist Will McWhinney, and musician David Dunn (Thompson, 1986, 1989; Brodsky, 1986). They have envisioned the HIV/AIDS phenomenon as a signal of the emergence of a new culture. They see the loss of membranal integrity as a signal of the loss of autopoetic unity analogous to the breaking down of boundaries at a global level between countries, ideologies, and disparate groups. Thompson views HIV/AIDS not simply as a chance infection but part of a larger cultural phenomenon and sees the pathogen not as an object but as heralding the need for living together characterized by a symbiotic relationship:

> AIDS could also signify an even greater "membrane" anomaly that calls upon us to reconceptualize the "nature" of the "self". . . . We may need to change our ideas of treatment to ones in which the immune system is "retuned" to new states of harmonic integration in which we learn to tolerate aliens by seeing the self as a cloud in a clouded sky and not as a lord in a walled-in fortress. (Thompson, 1989, p. 99)

The superconsciousness that McWhinney and Dunn (Brodsky, 1986) associate with HIV/AIDS is a collectivization that is dependent upon previous integration of all levels of consciousness in relation to a larger systemic awareness. The HIV/AIDS phenomenon is seen as an evolving cultural pattern of consciousness that transcends representation (separate entities defined by boundaries) and is nonlocal in nature.

Within this theoretical context, the present study was initiated to look at the evolving interactive pattern of persons who are HIV positive for evidence of changes consistent with expanding consciousness. Thus, the study questions were: What is the evolving pattern of selected persons diagnosed as HIV positive? How does the nurse interviewer interact with this pattern? Is this pattern a manifestation of health as expanding consciousness?

THE HEURISTIC RESEARCH PROCESS

This study was heuristic in nature, in that it was a "process of internal search through which one discovers the nature and meaning of experience" (Moustakas, 1990, p. 9). According to Moustakas, the researcher must have had a direct, personal encounter with the phenomenon being investigated. In this case the first author, who conducted the interviews, met that criterion. The interviewer sought to be an authentic, whole person as he engaged in the research process with the participants. The general elements of the process for collecting data were essentially the same as set out previously by Newman (1990, pp. 40, 41):

- Establish the mutuality of the process of inquiry
- Focus on the most meaningful persons and events in the interviewee's life
- Organize the data in narrative form and display it in a diagram as sequential patterns over time
- Share the interviewer's perception of the pattern with the interviewee and seek revision or confirmation.

The interviews were conducted at a community center for persons with HIV/AIDS in a large midwestern city. The director of the program assisted the interviewer in identifying potential participants, based on the participants being gay and having been identified as HIV positive. The purpose of the study was explained to them by the interviewer. If they agreed to participate, they were asked to sign an informed consent form that ensured their confidentiality and their right to withdraw from the study at any time. No one refused to participate in the study; however, one participant was unavailable for a follow-up interview and was not included in the pattern analysis that follows.

The resulting sample consisted of nine men ranging in age from 26 to 50 years old. Eight were Caucasian; one was both Native American and Caucasian. The time since HIV-positive diagnosis ranged from 6 months to 8 years; five men had an AIDS diagnosis, the time since diagnosis ranging from 1 month to 4 years. A Karnofsky performance status score was given to each participant; one scored 60, three scored 80, one scored 90, and 5 scored 100. T_4 cell counts ranged from 0 to 695. Six men were on antiretroviral medications. Five men were on antidepressant or antianxiety medications. Two men worked, one full time, one part time. Eight men did some type of volunteer work.

Interviews were conducted in a private room at the center and were tape-recorded. The procedure called for interviewing the participants twice, once to elicit their story of meaningful persons and events in their lives, and secondly to share the pattern diagram and obtain validation of the data. Immediately before the initial interview the purpose of the study was reviewed. Each participant was reminded that the interviewer was interested in having the participant tell his story. Then the 45- to 60-minute interview began with a directive statement such as "Tell me about the most meaningful persons or events in your life" and proceeded in a nondirective manner. The interviewer utilized active listening, clarification, reflection, self-disclosure, and intuitive hunches about what to say or ask; occasionally, more direct questions were needed if a participant was quiet, withdrawn, or depressed.

Following the first interview, the tape was transcribed and the transcript reviewed. The participant's own words were used in the development of a written narrative summary by putting key segments of data that highlighted meaningful occurrences and relationships into chronologic order. The data remained just as spoken; no interpretation was made. Natural breaks where a pattern shift occurred were noted. What evolved was a pattern of the whole made up of chronologic, sequential segments of the participant's story. A simple pattern diagram (modified from Newman, 1987) was created of each chronologic segment, which highlighted key people and events in relation to the participant. These were schematically identified by symbols that denoted mutual relationship, one-way relationship, broken or ended relationship, conflicted relationship, and unclear relationship.

Approximately a week later the interviewer met with the participant to share with him the diagram of his life as it unfolded in sequential configurations. No interpretation was made of the people or events in it. At this time the participant was asked to validate, clarify, or correct data from the interview, and, if necessary, the interviewer asked clarifying questions.

THE PATTERN OF THE WHOLE

The pattern of the whole emerged by spending time attending to the transcripts and summaries of the stories of these men and allowing the data to speak for themselves. Statements deemed important to the participants were clustered into themes, first for each of the participants and subsequently for the group.

The life stories of the participants revealed an evolving pattern of the whole. All but one man experienced *alienation* within their families while growing up, in the form of physical, emotional, or sexual abuse; oppression; or strictness. There was a definite *breaking away* from their family of origin through going to college, joining the military, finding jobs, moving out, or getting kicked out. All of the men experienced *cycles of aloneness and searching* through alcohol and/or drug use, sexual relationships, depression, suicide attempts or ideation, and/or multiple losses. Eventually, these cycles of aloneness and searching, coupled with having HIV/AIDS, led to a *turning point* at which they began to find new meaning in their lives.

The unfolding pattern can be visualized as a spiral of expanding consciousness, beginning in the center with the experiences of alienation, from which they broke away and moved into cycles of aloneness and searching and then gradually began to transcend their personal limitations as they dealt with the presence of HIV in their lives. Each person had a unique story to tell; yet each story shared the aspects of this unfolding pattern of expanding consciousness.

The following story, excerpted from the words of one of the participants, was selected as an exemplar of this pattern:

> [My parents] were strict . . . . not a lot of hugging with my father or mother. I was raised to be afraid of my father. I was terrified of this man. I had to say "yes, sir", "no, sir", "yes, ma'am", "no, ma'am." I'd get a smack in the face if I didn't do that. They gave me shelter, food, and they loved me the way they knew how. I think mom and dad were trying so hard to better their children from what they had; I think they forgot about the love.
>
> I took piano, classical, for 13 years. I sang. I took voice. I paid for those too. I was in all the plays in high school. I loved them. [My parents] came to one. [They said] a normal guy did not do stuff like that. My family wanted me to go to college after high school. I wanted to study music. I got accepted to the school of the arts. But mom and dad refused [to pay] my way to study anything that had to do with music. They said they'd pay my way toward college to study business. I gave in, like I always did to them. I wanted to get away from home. The day I was supposed to leave, I told them I was not going. I moved out of the house. We didn't speak for a while after that. I joined the Navy. And basically those 4 years I was on a ship seeing the world.
>
> [When I told my parents I was gay], my dad didn't cry, it's like he lost his best friend. It hurt him and it hurt me telling him too. My mom started screaming and crying: "Oh, dear God, why have you cursed me . . . I want to die." I got up and left and didn't speak to them for 7 or 8 months.
>
> One of the most meaningful events happened to me on my birthday [in] 1985 when I found out I was HIV positive. I remember that day very well. I got discharged [from the Navy] the same day—that's how I found out. From there everything started snowballing . . . getting into drugs and alcohol and everything. I had to tell my family. We grew farther and farther apart after that.
>
> I told Jeffrey [my lover]. I said "Well don't you think you should get tested?" And he never did . . . he was dead a year later. That's a major turning point in my life. It changed everything; my lover died, I built a wall

around me. I just didn't care. I was searching, and I think I'd been searching all these years for acceptance in my family, in the community, in myself. I really had no one to talk to when Jeffrey died, I had no one . . . to share the grief with. I didn't even get anything from my family.

The thing that really hurt me about this disease in the past few years is discrimination that I've had because I was HIV positive. Whether it be from the gay community, the treatment that I went through for the first time, and losing my job. I lost a lot of my friends because they didn't want to associate with me. The reason I lost my job was because they found out I was HIV positive.

I woke up one Friday morning, not caring. I thought: what's the reason why . . . I keep trying and trying, I mean I'm gonna die eventually. People . . . already act like I'm dead. [I] went to the crack house . . . and just sat in front of the television set and started smoking crack. I didn't care . . . I really had no one, no one. And even then I thought God had probably abandoned me too.

[Two days later] I left the hotel and I went home to my apartment. I couldn't cry or anything. It was like I lost all my emotions, my feelings . . . I'd really come to the bottom.

Going through [chemical dependency] treatment . . . I learned that I had a lot of shame about being gay, being HIV. I had to deal with a lot of shame issues, abuse issues with the family, verbal and some physical abuse when I was growing up. I'm an alcoholic and a drug addict. That'll never change but I've been sober now for over a year and going on 2 months now. And that is the longest that I have ever been sober in over 13 years.

I'm shocked that I'm still here. I ask myself why a lot of times. I used to think that I really didn't deserve to be here. All my friends, a lot of them have died. It's going on 8 years. I feel very good but that can change too. Who knows? This disease, it's just you have no control over it. Of course I get scared about being HIV sometimes . . . but you know my faith and my higher power, God, Jesus, or whatever, I'm not afraid of dying . . . and I know that I won't be alone.

I really believe there's a reason why I've been here this long now. Whether it's been to sober up and really start learning and experiencing life depending on how long I have left. I'm not afraid to tell people that I'm HIV now. I'm learning to like myself . . . I'm not ashamed any more.

I've met new people up here. I'm on disability now. Like everything has been falling into place up here for me . . . and I'm associating with my gay friends and my HIV friends. I want to experience what time I have left, and who knows, I may have another 8 years, I don't know. I want to wake up in the morning and see the trees . . . see the leaves . . . things that I always took for granted. Hear the birds sing. Sit down with a friend and have a cup of coffee . . . and talk. And really listen to him and about his worries. What time I do have left, I want to finally live.

I'm finally close to [my parents] after all these years. And it's a shame though that I know a lot of it had to do with this HIV thing and me sobering up. We sit down and have a great conversation. They know that I'm gay and that I'm HIV. This past year, it's like I finally got a family. I always had one but I'm finally acknowledging the fact that I got one. And they're proud of me.

The story of this man highlights the pattern of the whole seen in the participants: physical and emotional abuse while growing up within his family (*alienation*); moving out of the house and joining the military (*breaking away*); using alcohol and crack, struggling with depression, losing his lover, job, and friends (*cycles of aloneness and searching*); and going through chemical dependency treatment, finding new friends, reconnecting with his family, appreciating life (*turning point and beyond*).

TURNING POINTS

Young's spectrum of the evolution of consciousness (Young, 1976) was helpful in addressing the patterns depicted in the stories of these men. Young has described how persons move through the initial bonds imposed by the dictates of others in the environment to a search for their own identity and control of their lives. Eventually, they reach a critical point at which they realize that the old rules don't work any more. The person is faced with a turning point, a choice point. The task is to figure out the new rules by which the person will transcend the limitation of the old ways, release the old self-centeredness, and move on to a vision that goes beyond the self and leads to the freedom and power of expanding consciousness. With the realization of self-limitation, there is transcendence to inner freedom and expansion.

Reed points out that transcendence of self and broadened life perspective occur when one is dealing with end-of-own-life issues (Reed, 1991). For the men in this study, there was a turning point associated with having HIV in their lives and the recognition of their own mortality. They had experienced deep losses, such as the death of a lover, termination of a job, a destroyed career, and the uncertainty and physical problems of living with HIV/AIDS. For most, this new seeing was gradual. While it gave life a new perspective, it was not without its difficult moments and struggles. These men were able to persevere and to live life more fully in the midst of painful pasts and uncertain futures. Here are examples from each of the participants (in addition to the previous exemplar case) of what they faced:

> If it wasn't for the fact that you're gonna die and . . . that I suffer physically every single day, I would say having AIDS was a very pleasant positive experience because it's changed me for the better emotionally, mentally, socially for the better. But to get to that state you have to go through something that destroys your life.

> In a way having AIDS is a blessing because it's got me to do things that I would not normally do . . . . And it slowed me down and got me to go, to do things I would not normally have the money nor the time [to do].

> I don't care if I die but as least if I die, the time that I have lived I made the best of it that I can. You know, maybe not all of my life, but at least I've done something to change, the best that I can change.

> I always had a fear of being identified as being gay. It was one of my worst fears. When I tested HIV positive . . . it really opened up my life. I'd probably be in the closet yet. I'm sure I would be. I never really looked at it [HIV] as bad—it was opening up a new life for the most part. It's more of an open door for me. It's also a door that's gonna end, close, you know. I go through these periods of time where everything is going fine, then . . . I keep on saying to myself let's get this over with.

> It is a big courage for me to get out; taking the steps to meet other members who are here [at the center] has been a real positive experience. I really have to give myself credit for how far I've come since December.

> Now 3 weeks after this . . . brutal diagnosis, I'm to the point now that it's not *my* diagnosis, it's *their* diagnosis. It's what they, in their medical profile, have to deal with. But it's not what I have to deal with. I know how I feel physically, I know what I am capable of physically. I can feel the effects of HIV but I can also feel the effects of being a vibrant, live person . . . . In the whole scheme of things, HIV . . . has its own benefit to the world. It's really forcing people to deal with profound issues.

Facing the turning points in their lives was not easy or pain-free. The learning of new rules, of new ways of being in the world, was pursued in the midst of the ups and downs of having HIV/AIDS in their lives. Although these men had experienced many life struggles, when HIV/AIDS came into the picture they were eventually able to form more consistent patterns of connection and reconnection, of relating to self, others, and their spiritual values. With HIV/AIDS the transcendence of self unfolded:

> Helping out around here [at the center], that gives me the feeling like I'm not just a piece of clay or something. I've met people here that I really care about. It's kind of family for me. That's bonding with people who share something, it's kind of a spiritual thing for me . . . . sharing and feeling, feeling good about myself and, you know, feeling compassion and love for my friends and other people. For me, I guess it's love.

> Church has helped a lot in living with this disease. Just knowing the people that I know now. . . . Helping people. Those are meaningful things in my life. Jesus and God and church are really important to me.

> I realize how important certain people have been (i.e., my brothers and sisters and family). The biggest part of my life is continuing to work, share, and to be happy.

The expanding consciousness associated with coming to grips with HIV/AIDS can be seen in the changing quality of these men's lives.

The changes included feeling good about themselves, being more in charge of their lives, opening up to a fuller expression of their own caring and sharing, taking advantage of opportunities in life they would have ignored before, and a deepening of their spirituality. They were facing the profound issues of living and dying in a meaningful way.

THE RESEARCH AS PRAXIS

This research method is praxis in the sense that the process itself is emancipatory for the participants at the time the research is occurring. In the second interview, the men gave varying degrees of affirmation about participating in the interviews and seeing their pattern diagram. For example, one man said:

> The representation is very good. It's amazing to see it on paper. You were able to get such clear definition, clearer than I would be able to put on paper myself . . . but clear enough where I see my life on a piece of paper.

Another felt the experience gave him a perspective on his life and all he had accomplished in spite of many obstacles:

> I guess seeing it laid out on paper here really makes it more concrete for me. I guess the interview was a learning experience. Mostly for the simple fact that a lot of this . . . I never wrote down. It's a good learning experience to see how you have it laid out. And seeing this, too, it really helps me to have to say that [I] should really take credit for what I've done. I like the approach you are using . . . . I can almost see my personality in the chart.

And another found that the process allowed him to appreciate his life and talk to his partner about concerns he had about HIV/AIDS:

> It has made me think about where my life is. It has given me an opportunity to raise the question with my current partner and to be able to freely talk about it [HIV]. I think that more people should have this kind of discussion whether it be for a study or any other way.

THE EXPERIENCE OF THE INTERVIEWER

The interviewer's experience is integral to the process of pattern recognition, which is largely a function of the viewer's ability to see. The interviewer was able to share in the intimate moments of the lives of the participants while at the same time increasing his self-awareness about living with HIV and the patterns of his own life. The following is an excerpt from the interviewer's journal, which was kept throughout the interviewing process:

> During the first few interviews I struggled with what my role should be. Was I supposed to get the participants to talk about particular events and persons? Was I supposed to get them to recognize their pattern? I soon realized that all I had to do was "be there" and listen, to have the participant speak about whatever came up in the moment. I needed to let go of thinking I had to lead the interview in a direction or make the pain better or fix a problem. The purpose of the interview was to hear the story, to allow a sense of the whole to emerge just as the person told it. While it was necessary at times to ask clarifying questions and encourage elaboration, it was more important to be truly present to the story with all its pain, sadness, joy, and bittersweetness, allowing it to unfold just as it was spoken. In contrast, in nursing practice, so often I come filled with what I think should happen because my clinical role usually concerns a problem or a role function which needs to be fulfilled.

What is going on in the mutual patterning of the interviewer and participant? The holographic model explains what happens during the interaction of two people: "the waves radiating from each person interacting with the other pattern and becoming an interference pattern that is part of each person's pattern" (Newman, 1986, pp. 70, 71). This interpenetration of energy fields is part of pattern recognition in which the contrast of different patterns helps enlighten the evolving pattern of the whole. The holographic metaphor was apparent in the following entries from the interviewer's journal.

I am opening myself to the feelings that I experience during the interviews, thinking that what arises in me is a reflection of what is arising in the other—a holographic reflection. The opposite is also true— what arises in them is a reflection of me.

The metaphor of the hologram kept coming back to me during the interviews. In my being present through silence and unconditional attention, I had a sense of being a holographic mirror where [the interviewee] could see himself and his patterns reflected in my listening. And he was a holographic mirror for my story without my even speaking it. A part of each of us is in the other. Just through this process as it was in its simplicity, I felt an appreciation for the whole of his life reflected in the story. My receptivity, my releasing any hidden agenda to have him talk about a particular thing, allowed me to be a vessel to contain his story.

HIV/AIDS AS EXPANDING CONSCIOUSNESS

The data of this study support the view that the experience of HIV/AIDS is a manifestation of expanding consciousness. The loss of membranal integrity associated with HIV/AIDS opens the person to suffering and physical deterioration and at the same time introduces greater sensitivity and openness to self and others. The men in this study moved from being separated, alienated individuals in search of their place and connection in life to more meaningful, authentic relationships with self and others.

The question of whether or not other researchers would have reached the same conclusions must be addressed. The selectiveness of the sample might be a factor, since the participants were volunteers who were involved in the activities of a community center for people with HIV/AIDS and might have been predisposed for a transformative experience. Yet, this situation does not negate that the transformative experience did occur and is potentially available to all. Another more compelling explanation from the viewpoint of the authors lies in the interactive nature of the heuristic process: The nurse who interviewed these men was able to embrace the paradoxical nature of their stories, both the joy and pain, the living and dying, in such a way that they could be open to their world, that is, not be separated from the whole of their experience. The nurse's understanding of the phenomenon of health as expanding consciousness was integral to the mutual pattern of interaction with these men. Although he clearly did not direct their stories, the interpenetration of their fields created a symbiotic environment in which the participants could see their disease and other disruptive events as one with the unfolding pattern of expanding consciousness of their lives.

REFERENCES

Belcher, A. E., Dettmore, D., & Holzemer, S. P. (1989). Spirituality and sense of well-being in persons with AIDS. *Holistic Nursing Practice, 3*(4), 16–25.

Brodsky, A. B. (Ed.). (1986). The manners of chaos: A conversation between W. McWhinney and D. Dunn. *International Synergy, 1,* 40–51.

Carson, V. B., & Green, H. (1992). Spiritual well-being: A predictor of hardiness in patients with AIDS. *Journal of Professional Nursing, 8*(4), 209–220.

Carson, V., Soeken, K. L., Shanty, J., & Terry, L. (1990). Hope and spiritual well-being: Essentials for living with AIDS. *Perspectives of Psychiatric Care, 26*(2), 28–34.

Gloersen, B., Kendall, J., Gray, P., McConnell, S., Turner, J., & Lewkowiez, J. N. (1993). The phenomena of doing well in people with AIDS. *Western Journal of Nursing Research, 15*(1), 44–58.

Hall, B. A. (1990). The struggle of the diagnosed terminally ill person to maintain hope. *Nursing Science Quarterly, 3*(4), 177–184.

Korniewicz, D. M., O'Brien, M. E., & Larson, E. (1990). Coping with AIDS and HIV. *Journal of Psychosocial Nursing, 28*(3), 14–21.

Moustakas, C. (1990). *Heuristic research.* Newbury Park, CA: Sage.

Newman, M. A. (1979). *Theory development in nursing.* Philadelphia: F. A. Davis.

Newman, M. A. (1986). *Health as expanding consciousness.* St. Louis: Mosby.

Newman, M. A. (1987). Nursing's emerging paradigm: The diagnosis of pattern. In A. M. McLane (Ed.), *Classification of nursing diagnosis: Proceedings of the seventh conference, North American Nursing Diagnosis Association.* St. Louis: Mosby.

Newman, M. A. (1990). Newman's theory of health as praxis. *Nursing Science Quarterly, 3*(1), 37–41.

Nokes, K. M., & Carver, K. (1991). The meaning of living with AIDS: A study using Parse's theory of man-living-health. *Nursing Science Quarterly, 4*(4), 175–179.

Ragsdale, D., & Morrow, J. R. (1990). Quality of life as a function of HIV classification. *Nursing Research, 39*(6), 355–359.

Reed, P. G. (1991). Toward a nursing theory of self-transcendence: Deductive reformulation using developmental theories. *Advances in Nursing Science, 13*(4), 64–77.

Sowell, R. L., Bramlett, M. H., Gueldner, S. H., Gritzmach, D., & Martin, G. (1991). The lived experience of survival and bereavement following death of a lover from AIDS. *Image, 23*(2), 89–94.

Thompson, W. I. (1986). The Sunday evening evolutionary times. *International Synergy, 1,* 21–27.

Thompson, W. I. (1989). *Imaginary landscape: Making worlds of myth and science.* New York: St. Martin's Press.

Young, A. M. (1976). *The reflexive universe: Evolution of consciousness.* San Francisco: Robert Briggs Assoc.

CHAPTER FIFTEEN

The Spirit of Nursing

Margaret A. Newman

IN AMERICAN SOCIETY, separation of church and state is such a pervasive force that it carries over into the worlds of science and health. Things of a spiritual nature are considered separate from matters of science, and health (read medicine) is a matter of science. Grounded in the traditions of medicine and science, I at first was hesitant to address the concept of spirituality in nursing. As is often the case, I was getting spirituality mixed up with religion. Yet the root meaning of "holy," "whole," and "heal" is the same; so it seems that religion and the health professions are both concerned with the wholeness of life and perhaps are not so separate as we have been persuaded to believe. What are we talking about when we talk about spirituality or spirit? The spirit of the earth, says Teilhard de Chardin (1971), is humanity. It follows then that human interaction encompasses a spiritual component. Human interactions concerning health are matters of concern and responsibility to nursing.

My view of health includes disease as a meaningful manifestation of the pattern of the whole and is based on the premise that life is an ongoing process of expanding consciousness (Bentov, 1978b; Newman, 1986). Each person is a manifestation of the pattern of consciousness of all that there is. Both the seen pattern of our bodies and the unseen pattern of our minds, feelings, and spirits are manifestations of an underlying pattern (Bohm, 1980). Developing consciousness is manifest in a rhythmic interplay of order and disorder and evolves in the direction of greater complexity, higher frequency of wave interaction, and greater interpenetration of energy fields.

When Bentov talked about these things, someone said to him that he was talking about religion. He said, no, he was talking about knowledge (Bentov, 1978a). Similarly when I talk about interacting at levels beyond the bodymind manifestations of ourselves, I am not talking about religion in the traditional sense. These ideas do not contradict traditional religious tenets, but they do not represent religion.

Needleman makes it clear that consciousness is not what we call thinking, that it is something higher, greater. He sees the purpose of our lives as becoming attuned to this higher consciousness and believes that "every discipline in one way or the other has to contribute to that" (Needleham, 1988, p. 5). Actually, it is not so much "higher" consciousness as it is more inclusive. It includes both positive and negative states. (The term "higher" is used in this article to mean the broader, more inclusive phenomenon.)

Fox asks all professionals, "Whom are you serving?" He exhorts professionals to a ministry of imagination (spirit) and calls for a transformation of the world from slavery and bondage to freedom and justice (Fox, 1983, pp. 261, 264).

The profession of nursing is in a unique position to assist persons in this transformation. A recent experience with a woman who received a diagnosis of cancer brought these points home to me. What came through loud and clear in the decisions that were confronting her were a feeling of being enslaved to the conclusions and recommendations of the physician and an accompanying heaviness of dread and fear. When she let go of those feelings and sensed into the situation from the vantage point of her own life from her own perspective, the feeling she experienced was one of taking responsibility for herself—her whole self, not just the part that was diseased—and she felt free and right about her action. The health care system often does not support that kind of freedom, but nurses who are themselves free can be present at critical points for people and open up the possibility of freedom of choice.

The choice points presented by health crises are opportunities to experience more fully the reality of the patterns of our lives. Our experience in the bodymind state proceeds through a process of binding and centering, through which we find our identity and place in this world (Young, 1976). Things work fairly well for a while, and then we come to a choice point. This is a point at which the things that have worked for us in the past do not work anymore. Often this is a confrontation with disease, disability, or loss. The task confronting us is to learn what rules do apply, the new rules. If we can discover the rules and move to the other side of the choice point, we begin to regain the freedom lost in the process of becoming bound and centered in determinate matter. People who are able to transcend their physical limitations function in a timeless, boundaryless (spiritual) dimension. So how do nurses facilitate this kind of freedom? Here are a couple of ways that I have found helpful.

PATTERN RECOGNITION

The first, consistent with the human interaction patterns that form the framework of the North American Diagnosis Association Taxonomy I, is to assist clients in the identification of the pattern of their interaction with the environment (McLane, 1987). One can begin with the present pattern of interaction: who the person relates to, how they relate, what is important to the person, what choices he or she makes, what activities he or she engages in, and so on. Old patterns of interaction may arise and may differ markedly from the present pattern. A diagram of the sequential patterns of interaction over the lifetime of the person may indicate where the person is in terms of the process of expanding consciousness (manifested in the quality and diversity of interaction with the environment) (Newman, 1987a,

1987b). Concentration on the present flow of interaction will reveal the crucial pattern and will suggest areas where attention is needed to remove blocks in or to facilitate energy flow.

Take, for example, a woman from my research (Mrs. T.) who was in cardiac rehabilitation for care following a myocardial infarction that occurred a year previously. When asked to describe the most meaningful persons or events in her life, she got caught up in her current conflict with her adult children. From her point of view, two of her children, the oldest daughter and the son, "went off the track" and "rejected the teachings of the church," which to her was a rejection of her teachings and values. She feels that she invested her life in the children and that they have not turned out right and, therefore, she is a failure. She feels her life was wasted. She wants the children to come back home, acknowledge that they were wrong, and live their lives in accordance with "God's will."

Mrs. T. never contacts her children or initiates any conversation, and when they contact her, she does not express verbally what she is feeling and pretends that everything is all right. She is aware that "something is lacking" in her life and repeated several times that she feels like "a squirrel in a cage." Her husband encourages her to initiate communication with, in particular, her oldest daughter, but she feels he is not supporting her in her beliefs and feelings. She thinks she is at a stalemate.

The pattern of interaction of Mrs. T. during her childhood and adolescence was one of relative isolation from her parents. Then she married, had three children, and devoted her life to homemaking and cooking for her family. For a period of time, she felt close to her family; but when the children became adults, their choices of life style and companions were unacceptable to her and in her mind were wrong because they were in conflict with values upheld by her church. She now feels like a failure, feels hurt by her children's rejection of her values, and is unable to communicate her feelings to them or to maintain an ongoing relationship with them. She feels as though she is going round in circles with no way out of her "cage."

A diagram of the pattern of her relationships would show blocks in her communicating and relating to her adult children and between her and her husband. The purpose of this process of pattern identification is to facilitate the client's insight regarding the pattern. It is the client's insight that will open up the possibilities of a different level of interaction. The nurse in this situation was able to help Mrs. T. see the pattern of interaction she had established; but at the same time of the interview, Mrs. T. did not see that she had any responsibility for, or could so anything about, the block in communication between her and her children. This interview was part of a study designed to identify and verify patients' patterns of interaction and was limited to two interviews: one to solicit data about meaningful persons and events and the second to verify the pattern identified. Therefore, it is not known what transpired following these interviews. But based on the experience of subjects in other studies, I would speculate that as Mrs. T. is able to assimilate the pattern that was identified, she will see new possibilities of interaction with her family (Jonsdottir, 1988; Moch, 1988).

SENSING INTO ONE'S OWN FIELD

The second activity that the nurse can engage in, to bring about attunement to higher consciousness, is the process of sensing into one's own being. This sensing is consistent with a holographic model of intervention, which is based on the premise that the world we live in functions like a hologram (i.e., each part contains information about the whole). Sensing into one's own field, then, gives information about the whole. In the case of a nurse interacting with a patient, the energy fields of the two interact and form a new pattern of interpenetration, spirit within spirit. Sensing into one's own field gives information about the patient via the wave interference pattern that represents the nurse-patient interaction. Verbalizing what is sensed in one's own field often communicates an empathic understanding of what is going on for the other person and facilitates the patient's getting in touch with himself or herself and thereby becoming attuned to the larger context.

This process of sensing into one's own field requires attention to one's inner experience and trusting that it is valid information about the present interaction. The woman with cancer referred to earlier shared with me her experience of bodily pain and fear while telling members of her family about the diagnosis of cancer that she had received. As she described this interaction, I had a visual picture of her as the "sink" into which all of the fear of her family was flowing, and from her description of previous interactions with her family, I sensed that this pattern of interaction was true for other situations. The difference here was that, previously, she was the strong member who could absorb the fear. In this situation, she was the vulnerable member and was pained by the contradiction she was feeling between her own truth and the fear she was getting from her family. I related my "observation" of the sink to her and she indicated that if felt right for her experience. Her bodily sensation was signaling the incompatibility of the incoming energy from family members with her own energy, and she sensed the need to reverse the flow or otherwise alter the pattern of interaction.

To learn to do this, one has to be committed to "standing in the center of one's truth" (Arguelles, 1987) (i.e., being able to sense and communicate whatever is true for oneself in the moment). One way to start is to follow Gendlin's procedures for focusing (Gendlin, 1978). This process involves concentration on the feelings one is aware of in the body, such as a heaviness or pain in the heart or in other specified areas, or something far more diffuse. The task is to concentrate on that feeling until the identification of the feeling coincides with the deeper, nonverbal, message of the body. When this congruence is reached, there is usually a total relaxing shift that occurs in the body and a freeing of energy for transformation. As one becomes sensitive to one's own thoughts, feelings, and pictures (and learns to trust them), one will become adept at doing this quickly, instantly when interacting with another; one's own field becomes a reflective mirror of the interpenetration of the two fields.

The task of the nurse is to facilitate the patient's insight into his or her own pattern. The question that echoes over the years is, "But what does the nurse do in relation to the pattern?" The action indicated will become apparent only as the pattern becomes apparent, and the action is relevant only to the "truth" discovered by clients as they find the center of their truth and discover the new rules that apply to their situations.

Martin describes the process as a rhythmical coming together and moving apart of the client and the nurse (Martin, 1985). She sees the process as occurring in three steps: (1) meeting, (2) forming shared consciousness, and (3) moving apart. The meeting occurs because the patterns of the nurse and the patient have some congruence and there is a mutual attraction. The forming of shared consciousness requires recognition of the whole of each person and sharing to form a connection, the feeling of "clicking" with another person, or being "in synch." The nurse needs to be fully present, "100 percent observer and 100 percent participant," for the meeting "to gel" and "form a new pattern of the same substance." The nurse "stays clear" and "waits, waits, waits" in the resonating process while attending to the words, colors, skin, muscles, breathing, messages, images, and spirit of the patient:

To earth
To centre
To nest the spirit
To feel the skin
To think/see clearly
To reach for contact

Believing it comes,
Is 'to just know'
. . . that healing happens
In the contact (Martin, 1985)

Moving apart occurs as the client is able to center without being connected to the nurse. It does not occur all at once. The client and nurse move apart, then reconnect and move apart again, repeating the process until the client can see clearly.

The essence of nursing is not doing or manipulating but is being open to whatever arises in the interaction with the client. It is being fully present, with an unconditional acceptance of the client's experience. The nurse offers his or her whole self so that the client can resonate with an authentic person. The nurse is like a tuning fork through which the client can begin to resonate with the consciousness of the universe.

REFERENCES

Arguelles, J. (1987). *Mayan new year: Countdown to harmonic convergence.* Santa Fe: Doorways. Audio cassette.

Bentov, I. (1978a). Post-conference workshop on new dimensions of consciousness, Sufi Order in the West. New York, November 20.

Bentov, I. (1978b). *Stalking the wild pendulum.* New York: Dutton.

Bohm, D. (1980). *Wholeness and the implicate order.* London: Routledge & Kegan Paul.

Fox, M. (1983). *Original blessing.* Santa Fe: Bear.

Gendlin, E. T. (1978). *Focusing.* New York: Everest.

Jonsdottir, H. (1988). *Health patterns of clients with chronic obstructive pulmonary disease.* Master's thesis. University of Minnesota, Minneapolis, MN.

Martin, Margaret. (13 November 1985). Letter to author.

McLane, A. M. (Ed). (1987). *Classification of nursing diagnoses, proceedings of the seventh conference, North American Nursing Diagnosis Association, 9–12 March 1986.* St. Louis: Mosby.

Moch, S. D. (1988). *Health in illness: Experiences with breast cancer.* Ph.D. dissertation. University of Minnesota, Minneapolis, MN.

Needleman, J. (1988). Spirituality and the intellect. In *Thinking allowed. Institute of Noetic Sciences special report* (p. 5). Sausalito, CA: Institute of Noetic Sciences.

Newman, M. A. (1986). *Health as expanding consciousness.* St. Louis: Mosby.

Newman, M. A. (1987a). Nursing's emerging paradigm: The diagnosis of pattern. In A. M. McLane (Ed.), *Classification of nursing diagnoses. Proceedings of the seventh conference, North American Nursing Diagnosis Association, 9–12 March 1986.* St. Louis: Mosby.

Newman, M. A. (1987b). Patterning. In M. Duffy & N. J. Pender (Ed.), *Conceptual issues in health promotion. Proceedings of a Wingspread Conference, Racine, Wisc., 13–15 April 1987.* Indianapolis: Sigma Theta Tau

Teilhard de Chardin, P. (1971). *Activation of energy.* New York: Harcourt Brace Jovanovich.

Young, A. M. (1976). *The reflexive universe: Evolution of consciousness.* San Francisco: Robert Briggs.

PART FOUR

Integrating Theory, Education, and Practice

The declaration in 1965 that baccalaureate education should be the basis for professional education in nursing was a step in the right direction, but not enough. The major paradigm then guiding nursing education, licensure, and practice was based on the medical model. We had some pre-paradigmatic knowledge of nursing science at that time, but efforts to transform nursing education and practice by integrating this knowledge did not make a noticeable difference, such was the power of the medical paradigm.

With the 1965 declaration, and the advent of associate degree programs to prepare nursing technicians, we embarked on a continuing effort to differentiate professional nursing from technical nursing, without much success except to say that professional nursing was based on a broader and more complex view of the phenomenon. As the focus of the discipline became clearer, however, it became also clear that what we have been regarding as professional nursing is based on a holistic view of the client's health experience and what we have considered primarily technical nursing is based on the application of medical technology. *The difference was a matter of paradigm: person-oriented care vis-á-vis disease-oriented care.* Since most nurses have functioned within hospitals, which are dominated by the medical paradigm, the bulk of nursing practice has been medical technology.

In the last decade, differentiated practice models have been developed to distinguish between professional and technical care, but they have not, for the most part, recognized the paradigm dilemma. What I offer takes into consideration this dilemma and the difference in paradigms. It includes a connecting link to provide nursing leadership for the translation of medical directives into person-oriented care. The roles of the tri-level model correspond, first, to the nursing paradigm, second, to technology emanating from the medical paradigm, and third, to the transformation of medical technology to a holistic paradigm. The roles are related to the three predominant levels of preparation for nursing practice; however, changes in the curricula of these programs are needed to facilitate a better fit with the intended practice mode, and thus provide the basis for an *integrated* practice.

The changes in health care delivery brought about by prospective payment systems have forced a more intense emphasis on medical technology within shorter periods of hospitalization, further diminishing the professional focus of nursing in hospitals. At the same time, the need for nursing coordination to bridge the acute-to-chronic phases of patient care across health care settings has become equally intense. This need increased opportunities for nurses to function in authoritative roles stemming from the nursing paradigm in direct relation to clients *whenever and wherever* the need arose and allowed for the emergence of nurse case managers. The practice of the nurse case management group at Carondelet St. Mary's in Tucson, Arizona, for example, reflects the philosophy and focus of the discipline of nursing and serves as a model for nurses as primary care providers.

In order to prepare the kind of authoritative professional practitioner that nursing is capable of, and that society needs, we need a curriculum that goes beyond baccalaureate education. Master's programs have been expanding to fill this need but represent a piecemeal approach to professional education and fall short of a clearly professional, post-baccalaureate degree comparable to those offered in other professional disciplines. Two decades ago Rozella Schlotfeldt called for a professional doctorate in nursing and later developed the first such program at Frances Payne Bolton School of Nursing at Case Western Reserve University. My own inspiration for such a program came from Ruth Neil Murry, then dean of nursing at the University of Tennessee in Memphis. Progress has been slow, but now there are three such programs.*

These issues—the entry of the nurse as a primary care provider, and a truly nursing model of professional education—are the primary issues for the profession as we move into the 21st century.

---

* University of Colorado and Rush University, in addition to Case Western Reserve. Two other programs are being developed.

CHAPTER SIXTEEN

Professionalism: Myth or Reality

Margaret A. Newman

HAVE WE AS nurses deluded ourselves regarding our professionalism? We call ourselves professionals and interminably defend the development of our profession. Yet at the present time, we are still largely unsuccessful in actualizing a distinction between professional nursing and its technical counterpart. We have the mission, knowledge, and commitment for a vital professional service to society. Why then is it not a reality?

A professional relationship involves a direct connection in the form of an informal contract between the professional and the client for an identifiable service in a particular area of expertise. It is not bound by place or time. It requires knowledgeable judgment in a specific area. The client makes the ultimate decision whether or not the relationship occurs and is maintained.

A technical role involves the performance of repetitive tasks prescribed by and under the surveillance of a professional authority. The performance of these tasks requires specific knowledge and judgment. The place and time of the performance of these tasks is determined by the professional or institutional authority. Persons performing these tasks are readily exchangeable.

Reprinted with permission from *The Nursing Profession: Turning Points* (pp. 49–52), edited by N.L. Chaska, C.V. Mosby, St. Louis. Copyright by Mosby-Year Book, 1990.

The law defining professional nursing incorporates a dependent function, the ultimate authority for which rests with the medical profession. Medical technology comprises the major portion of the practice of nursing in hospitals. Observation of the work of hospital nurses reveals primarily the performance of delegated medical treatments and observations with little or no *specific nursing* connection to the patients.

This was not always so. In the early history of nursing, nurses functioned relatively independently in direct relationships to individuals regardless of whether or not the individual had a diagnosed disease. Increasingly, however, nursing became more dependent on medical authority and hospitals for its practice. The momentum of our recent history has been to widen the dependent path by expanding the performance of tasks aimed at the diagnosis and treatment of disease (Orlando, 1987).

As I talk to nurses about their current practice (Newman & Autio, 1986), I am forced to conclude that the fulfillment of a professional role in nursing is largely a myth. Schlotfeldt (1987) too concludes that "nursing remains essentially an other-directed and controlled occupation, rather than a self-directed profession."

A MATTER OF PARADIGM

Bruner (1986) suggests that myth serves as a substitute or filter for experience. Nurses who are committed to taking good care of patients and who work hard and are skilled in what they do are convinced that they are functioning as professionals, in spite of the fact that their work more clearly fits the definition of technical practice. These attributes—human compassion, dedication, and technical expertise—are *essential but not sufficient* to characterize the whole of nursing professional practice. We have debated the issue of professional vis-á-vis technical for at least a quarter of a century, with little resolution. Recently I realized with astonishing clarity that the issue is not primarily one of professional versus technical! The issue is one of *different paradigms of practice:* person-oriented care in contradistinction to disease-oriented care.

An editorial by Mary Mallison (1987) called for a recognition of the need for different types of practitioners with different types of education and for both types of practitioners to respect the abilities of the other. A reasonable exhortation. Why haven't we been able to accomplish it? In order to do so we need to recognize that the barrier to valuing the role and education of each other is the fact that the different roles and educational programs emphasize different paradigms, *different world views.* The predominant practice perspective derives from the paradigm of health as the absence of disease, a paradigm in which the "battle" against disease is uppermost and the practice mode is one of dominance and control. The person-oriented health paradigm, espoused by the nursing profession, places personal meaning and quality of life at the forefront and requires a practice mode of collaboration and mutuality. When one is viewing the world from one side, it is difficult to imagine, much less value, the view from the other side.

Schlotfeldt (1987) sees "the perspective within which nurses view their world of work and inquiry" as crucial to the future of nursing. She points out that we are agreed that nursing's mission is the optimizing of persons' health. But there is where the agreement ends: Is this mission for all persons or just for those being treated for medical problems?

Divergent views on this issue indicate different paradigms of health. And different paradigms of health require different types of technology. If the institution is ruled by the medical paradigm, activities within that paradigm are the ones that will be honored and rewarded. Nurses functioning primarily in the medical model are operating in the currently more powerful paradigm: those functioning primarily in the nursing model are addressing concerns that are viewed as nonessential extras by the prevailing paradigm. The "anti-education" bias that Mallison (1987) refers to among practicing nurses is more a function of conflicting paradigms than of educational status. If it is important that nursing concern itself with both paradigms, then at least we should know what paradigm directs the practice.

Nursing roles within the hierarchy of medically oriented institutions are under the authority of medicine and the institutional administration. In the past, some of the professional priorities of nursing were integrated in this role. The current emphasis on cost-effectiveness within institutions dominated by the medical paradigm accentuates the priority of the medical regimen in the delivery of care, and nursing practice within this system is diminished as nursing priorities fall by the wayside.

AN OPPORTUNITY TO ACTUALIZE
PROFESSIONAL NURSING

The authority of a profession lies in its knowledge. The professional role requires *a direct relationship with the client on an ongoing basis*. It permits relative autonomy in decision making based on the knowledge of the professional discipline.

The nursing void created by dominance of the medical model is making room for a new nursing practitioner* who is responsible directly to patients for coordinating their continuing care wherever they might be—in the hospital, at home, or in other health care sites. The functions of this nurse are not new, but the designated position makes it possible to actualize the essence of nursing in a direct connection to clients on an ongoing basis, regardless of setting, for as long as the

---

* This position has been referred to alternately as a patient care coordinator, continuing care coordinator, and case manager. Although the case manager title has gained more recognition, the term *case* connotes an impersonal approach and the term *manager* connotes one-sided dominance, both of which meanings are antithetical to the person-centered collaborative approach of the nursing paradigm.

client has a need for nursing care—a truly professional role that stems from the nursing paradigm.

The impetus for this continuing care role is the realization, both public and professional, of today's general lack of personalized care and the tremendous gap in patients' ability to care for themselves after hospitalization. Expanding hospital corporate structures now include the full spectrum of health care services, with increasing emphasis on home and ambulatory care; this expanded structure makes it possible to employ nurses in positions that span the various care settings. Private insurance companies have moved ahead to provide reimbursement of long-term care, and governmental support will probably not be far behind. Professionally educated nurses are well prepared to relate to clients in ways consistent with the emerging paradigm of health and to collaborate with clients and other health professionals in the coordination of their care.

There is a common stereotype of technology as inhuman and concerned primarily with machines and techniques. This is the stereotype that nurses tend to reject. A more illuminating view of technology is stated by Eisler (1987) as "the use of both tools or techniques *and our bodies and mind to achieve human-defined goals*" (p. 55). The emphasis here is on human. This definition has meaning for nursing technology as we interact with clients on a human-to-human level and use ourselves as well as the knowledge and techniques at our disposal to assist clients in their health-related goals. A paradigm shift toward a collaborative model of practice based on person-centered patterns of health *is occurring,* and when it establishes itself as the prevailing paradigm, medical technology will assume its place as an alternative within the whole, rather than as the primary focus. A shift in paradigm does not discard the old knowledge; it transforms it by viewing it from another perspective. If we are clear on the perspective of the nursing paradigm, we can transform medical technology within the larger context of nursing.

We are at a turning point in the development of our profession. During the early first phase of our development, the knowledge of our practice was derived through intuition and qualities of human caring. As we moved into the second stage, the medical paradigm dominated the education of nurses. The emphasis was on knowledge about disease, its recognition, and treatment. Emphasis was on finding out what was wrong and taking action to remedy the situation. The responsibility for performance of a large aspect of medical technology was delegated to and accepted by nursing. At the same, nursing educators recognized the importance of knowledge about health per se and about patients as persons. In the current stage, as the transition to a person-oriented health curriculum takes priority, we are faced with conflict because the practice world is still dominated by the medical paradigm, and we are uncertain how the transformation will take place.

UNITED DIVERSITY

We need to unite as a profession. We have bemoaned the confusion inherent in the statement that "a nurse is a nurse is a nurse." Now is the time to recognize the core of nursing in the various roles that nurses perform. Nurses have a perspective on health that is important and have a responsibility to society to be involved in the planning and coordinating of the continuing care of individuals and their families. Nurses need also to be involved in the direct day-to-day care, which incorporates medical and nursing technology. Nurses need to be involved in the organization and implementation of this care wherever it occurs. But the same nurse cannot do it all. One nurse plans and coordinates on a continuing long-term basis; another nurse organizes and coordinates the care in immediate short-term settings; and another nurse provides the day-to-day direct care in both institutional and home settings. The execution of these three roles requires different types of expertise and different educational preparation. There is some consensus that the coordinator role, which spans institutions and settings, requires master's level preparation;* the organizer/supervisor role within a specific setting, a baccalaureate degree; and the direct care provider, an associate degree (Stull, Pinkerton, Primm, Smeltzer, & Walker, 1986).

In the past we have practiced an all-or-nothing approach in handling these responsibilities. Now we need to recognize the essentials of each of the above roles and the aspects that can be performed more effectively by each. This approach involves delegation, not in the traditional sense from top to bottom, but in the sense of shared and differentiated responsibility.

There is great dissatisfaction with the old system of health care and a need to burst into a new organization. Transformation will involve moving from a dominator model to a partnership model. The practice of nursing is not, as Mechanic and Aiken (1986) so ably put it, "the soft underbelly" of medicine but the mind and heart that makes transformation of the health experience possible.

CONCLUSION

Nursing practice is riddled with the problem of mixed paradigms. The predominant paradigm, health as absence of disease, is embraced by the medical model and incorporates characteristics of a paradigm of patriarchy such as dominance, power, efficiency, and control. The nursing model embraces a paradigm of dynamic patterning of relationships. It incorporates the feminine principles of caring, cooperation, collaboration, and mutuality. Nursing has been caught in a catch-22 situation. We have been mesmerized by the myth of professionalism in the status quo and have allowed our energy to be dissipated both in support

---

* A master's degree in nursing is generally agreed upon as preparation for this case manager role; however, I continue to take the position that a professional doctorate (ND) is the preferred degree (See Chapter 20).

of and opposition to the medical paradigm. It is time to recognize the values and directives of the nursing paradigm and move into the reality of our professional responsibility.

REFERENCES

Bruner, J. (1986). *Actual minds, possible worlds.* Cambridge: Harvard University Press.

Eisler, R. (1987). The chalice and the blade: Technology at the turning point. *International Synergy, 2*(1), 54–63.

Mallison, M. (1987). Must we be divided by degree? *American Journal of Nursing, 87,* 763.

Mechanic, D., & Aiken, L. H. (1986). Social science, medicine and health policy. In L. H. Aiken & D. Mechanic (Eds.), *Applications of social science to clinical medicine and health policy.* New Brunswick, NJ: Rutgers University Press.

Newman, M., & Autio, S. (1986). *Nursing in a prospective payment system health care environment.* Minneapolis: University of Minnesota School of Nursing.

Orlando, I. J. (1987). Nursing in the 21st century: Alternate paths. *Journal of Advanced Nursing, 12,* 405–412.

Schlotfeldt, R. M. (1987). Resolution of issues: An imperative for creating nursing's future. *Journal of Professional Nursing, 3,* 136–142.

Stull, M. K., Pinkerton, S., Primm, P., Smeltzer, C., & Walker, M. K. (1986). Entry into practice roundtable. *Current Concepts in Nursing, 1*(1), 2–7, 10–12.

CHAPTER SEVENTEEN

Nursing in a Changing Health Care System

Margaret A. Newman

Sharon Autio

A MAJOR SHIFT in health care financing has occurred in response to the rising costs of health care services. In an effort to control Medicare expenditures, Congress passed legislation in 1983 changing the method of hospital reimbursement from a cost-based retrospective system to a prospective payment system based on diagnosis related groupings (DRGs). Hospital costs exceeding the DRG payment are absorbed by the hospital; costs less than the designated amount yield a surplus for the hospital. In Minnesota other forms of health care financing, specifically health maintenance organizations (HMOs) and self-insured employers, have similar payment systems and it is anticipated that some form of prospective payment will soon pervade the entire spectrum of health care financing. Minnesota Senator Durenberger has said, "We want to prospectively price not only Medicare services but eventually Medicaid and all personal health care services regardless of provider or setting."

Excerpted from Newman, M. & Autio, S. (1986). Nursing in the world of DRGs and prospective payment. *CURA Reporter* 16(5), University of Minnesota Center for Urban and Regional Affairs.

One of the results of implementing the prospective payment system is shortened hospital stays and more intensified home nursing and medical care. Under the guidelines developed by Medicare, and by many of the HMOs, patients cannot be admitted to hospitals without pre-admission screening to determine whether or not the hospitalization is eligible for reimbursement. In addition, the length of hospitalization is specified according to the patient's diagnosis; extensions of hospitalization beyond the specified length of stay must be approved by the funding agency. It is generally agreed that under the new system patients are more acutely ill both when they are admitted to the hospital and when they are discharged. This intensifies the work of the hospital nursing staff and transfers a large portion of the acute care of the patient to the home. These changes are bringing about two issues of major concern to citizens of Minnesota: limited access to hospital care and increased individual responsibility for home care.

The research project reported here was designed to describe and interpret current patterns of health care under the prospective payment system in representative sites in the Twin Cities metropolitan area. Recommendations are made for nursing practice under the new system and for consumer access to health care.

METHODS OF THIS STUDY

Three hospitals and their satellite outpatient operations were chosen as representative of health care delivery in the Twin Cities metropolitan area. Hospitals are the major providers of acute care services and continue to employ the majority of registered nurses. The three chosen were an urban public tertiary-care institution, an urban private multihospital system facility, and a private rural community hospital.

Interviews were conducted during the 1985–86 academic year with three levels of nursing personnel at each of the hospitals: nursing administrators, head nurses, and staff nurses. Key individuals were chosen for the interviews. The initial interview, with directors of nursing, used a semi-structured questionnaire format to obtain general demographic data on the hospital and its operations. These administrators were asked to identify head nurses whom they considered representative and head nurses, in turn identified staff nurses to be interviewed. Interviews with head nurses and staff nurses were essentially unstructured although key questions were asked of both groups. They were asked to describe the current pattern of nursing care delivery on their respective units, their particular role in care, and things that they liked or disliked about their work. The content of the interviews was summarized and shared orally in a meeting with the nurses at each site so that its accuracy could be verified. The summaries were then analyzed and compared, and a synthesis of predominant themes compiled.

Interviews were also conducted with nurses in home care, nurses employed by HMOs, and nurses in alternative care models. The director of a public health nursing organization, the director of a freestanding corporate agency, and the director of a hospital-based department of home health care were asked to identify their current home care offerings, how consumers in need of home care gain access to their services, how their programs are staffed, and how they are reimbursed. A summary was sent to each person interviewed for verification or correction.

Nurses employed by three of the HMOs in the Twin Cities area were interviewed and asked to describe the current and future roles for registered nurses within their organizations as well as their impressions of the changes occurring in the health care industry.

And finally, five consumers were interviewed either in person or by telephone and asked to describe their experiences with obtaining health care services and to discuss any problems they may have confronted with gaining access to the health care system.

FINDINGS OF THE TWIN CITIES SURVEY

Nursing in the Hospital

Patients who come into the hospital are sicker than they were before the prospective payment system was implemented, and they go home sooner. This is because of the approval mechanisms required by Medicare and HMO regulations, first in terms of pre-admission screening and second in terms of permissible length of hospitalization in relation to medical diagnosis. The effect on nursing has been to bring about an increased density and intensity of workload in the medical regimen to be carried out. Little time or energy is left for attending to the psychosocial aspects of illness and hospitalization or for teaching patients and their families what they can expect and how to care for themselves. The emphasis is on the medical treatments and observations that must be done while the patient is in the hospital. Preparation for discharge must begin as soon as the patient is admitted and is usually performed by the head nurse, a special discharge planner, or a person designated by the HMO to carry out this function.

Generally the way in which patient care is assigned is described as total patient care, meaning that the staff nurse is responsible for the total nursing care of assigned patients for an eight-hour shift. Total patient care includes administration of prescribed medical treatments, observation of the patients' conditions, and assistance with activities of daily living. The staff nurse's assignment is made by the charge nurse or in some instances by the charge nurse on the previous shift. A patient may have the same nurse assigned to her or him over the period of hospitalization, but there is no built-in mechanism for assuring continuity or consistency of assignments. The nurse's preferences or other work assignments may be the determining factors. If Licensed Practical Nurses (LPNs) are part of the staff, their assignments are similar to those of the Registered Nurses (RNs). Nursing aides, when available, are used as assistants to the RNs and LPNs to perform household tasks and run errands.

The head nurses' responsibilities are divided between personnel management and patient management. They have more responsibilities than they have time to complete, but when asked, they do not want to give up either focus of activity. The head nurses feel that they could fulfill their responsibilities better if they had greater control and flexibility in their own use of time.

The directors of nursing expressed a preference for an increased percentage of RNs on their staff. The current RN complement ranges from 69 to 88 percent. This is consistent with the national trends. The Twin Cities directors prefer RNs over LPNs because their greater preparation gives them more diverse abilities so that they can function anywhere in the hospital when additional staff are needed. Staff are encouraged to be generalists so that they can be reassigned if necessary to meet the hospital's needs. Often staff nurses do not know where they will be working until they arrive at the hospital, at which time they are assigned to a unit other than their home base. RNs are viewed as being very versatile, and with the increasing percentage of all RN staffs, they are asked to assume more non-nursing tasks (such as transporting patients, cleaning equipment and serving trays), an aspect of their job that they identified as objectionable.

Most of the nursing staff do not work full time. The reason for this appears to be both the fluctuating needs of the hospital and the extenuating demands of the job. When the census is low, administration "requests" that nursing staff take "voluntary" days off. When the census is high, staff are asked to work extra days and may be reassigned to other units. The result is that the staff who are employed are working at an intense pace and may be working in an area not of their choosing. Staff indicate that hospital nursing is too physically and emotionally demanding to work full time, that they need the extra time off in order to maintain their own health. Because of their part-time status and the variation in the number of days worked each pay period, their income varies accordingly. Some staff, in spite of the inconvenience of not knowing when these "days off" will occur or how much their salary will be that month, say that they don't mind the setup because it "gives them more time with their families;" but they acknowledge that this arrangement is difficult for single persons or heads of households because they can never be sure of a guaranteed income and have quite a balancing act to perform in terms of child care. The difficulty of part-time status was one of the issues of the 1984 nurses' strike in the Twin Cities. The trend toward part-time employment of nurses is accelerating in several major cities and Minneapolis-St. Paul (with 65 percent working part-time) has the second highest part-time complement in the country.

The dissatisfactions expressed by nursing staff focused on performance of non-nursing tasks, lack of control of their work schedule, and lack of involvement in administrative decisions affecting their work situation. These factors have been noted repeatedly in other analyses of nursing practice settings and in spite of them, most of the nurses interviewed expressed a high level of dedication to their work.

There is little opportunity for advancement of nurses in the clinical role. Advancement takes the form of moving up in the nursing administration hierarchy.

Nursing in the Home

In response to the increasing demand for home care after hospitalization and for assistance with health problems of the elderly, both of the private hospitals surveyed had established home care departments. The urban public hospital contracts with a public health nursing organization (PHNO) for home care services.

Staffing in the PHNO differs considerably from that in the hospital-based home care departments. The PHNO has a full-time staff of public health nurses (usually baccalaureate degree preparation) and home health aides. Some of the nurses have graduate preparation in clinical nursing specialization. The agency offers specialized team care for high risk families, terminally ill patients, and patients needing acute intravenous antibiotic treatment. The average case load ranges from twenty-five to sixty clients.

Both of the private home care units are staffed primarily with part-time RNs and additional on-call RNs and home health aides. Some of the on-call nurses are hospital-based staff who are used for home care if needed when the inpatient census is low. In one of the private home care units, nurses function as case managers and rotate twenty-four hour on-call responsibility.

All three agencies offer skilled nursing care that qualifies for Medicare and similar third-party reimbursement. In accordance with Medicare regulations, the need for nursing care in the home is dependent on medical necessity and must have a physician's approval. Home care nurses are responsible for assessing patients' needs for home care but are unable to authorize that care without a physician's approval.

The second major need, extended long-term care of chronically-ill patients, does not qualify for Medicare benefits. This need is growing rapidly with the increasing needs of the elderly. Both private home care units offer extended home care but third-party reimbursement is not readily available and most patients must be able to pay directly for these services. In some instances when patients are unable to pay, they are referred to publicly-financed home care agencies.

Patients are usually seen within twenty-four hours of discharge from the hospital, though a time lag may result from insufficient information about the client's health care needs. Considerable time is spent in determining reimbursement for services and detailed documentation of services must be maintained to satisfy third-party payors.

Although many patients in the home receive medical treatments requiring technical expertise, the directors interviewed feel that the major emphasis of home care is on teaching patients and families how to care for themselves. They see nurses as being the coordinators and facilitators of health care. Characteristics deemed important in home care nurses are ability to function autonomously, ability to assimilate and personalize medical care to patients' situations, and good communication and interpersonal skills. Within this context, they see a major need for professional supervision of unskilled care on an ongoing basis.

Nursing in HMOs

Nurses are employed in several roles within health maintenance organizations: patient care coordinators, direct providers, pre-admission screeners/utilization reviewers, and corporate executives.

Patient care coordinators, or case managers, continuously monitor the patient's condition, collaborate with other health professionals in planning the patient's care, and provide information to the patient and family regarding available resources. The patient care coordinator interviewed saw her major responsibility as assisting with discharge planning for an average caseload of thirty to forty patients per week. Most of these patients were elderly. She expressed great satisfaction in this role, citing the autonomy with which she functions and the contact with patients and their families as the most important, satisfying aspect of her work.

Direct care providers are employed with patients in a clinical situation. They vary in levels of preparation and roles. Certified nurse midwives, usually with a master's degree, are responsible for a specific case load and carry twenty-four hour responsibility for their clients. Obstetricians are involved only if complications occur in the pregnancy.

Nurse practitioners, either master's prepared or otherwise certified, are each responsible to a particular physician. Their responsibilities differ according to the clinic and specialty area in which they work. For example, an adult nurse practitioner may be responsible for treating certain minor illnesses and monitoring clients with chronic diseases. Nurse practitioners in the obstetrics/gynecology area are responsible for routine examinations, including Pap smears.

Pediatric nurse practitioners monitor well babies and administer immunization medications as ordered.

LPNs are employed to assist physicians by preparing patients for physical examinations, following through with specific diagnostic tests or procedures, administering prescribed medications, and performing household tasks.

Nurses who function as pre-admission screeners interact primarily with physicians rather than clients. Their major role is in utilization review during hospitalization. They monitor the patient's care to assess medical necessity and have the authority to levy financial restraints on providers who do not comply.

Other nurses are responsible for authorizing home health care. They make an initial assessment visit with a member of the contracting agency to determine whether or not the case qualifies for payment. This role contains aspects of both case management and utilization review.

In one HMO, nurses also function in a triage capacity by answering a sixteen hour phone line available to members for information about their health care questions.

A number of nurses hold upper management positions in operations and marketing. These nurses usually hold dual graduate degrees in nursing and business administration.

Consumer Concerns

The problems consumers face in the current health care system are problems of access to the system, information about various alternatives for health care and transfer from facility to facility or professional to professional within the system. A case example will serve to illustrate this point.

> The patient, an 89-year-old man, was living at home with his wife of approximately the same age. He was enrolled in an HMO and was a veteran.

He had two adult children, a son and a daughter who was a nurse. While the daughter was out of town, Mr. X., a known borderline diabetic, experienced some symptoms of a stroke but was not incapacitated. The next day he fell. The son called the clinic and they instructed him to bring his father to the hospital outpatient department. Diagnostic tests confirmed the stroke, but the physician said there was nothing to be done and that the family should take "good care" of him at home. When the daughter came home, almost a week later, she noticed that Mr. X was having difficulty with his speech, memory loss, and difficulty walking. He was eating often, sleeping, and very thirsty. She wondered if his diabetes was out of control.

The daughter called the physician, but his response was that she was "handling things fine." Her father became increasingly thirsty, irritable, hungry, and weak. Finally she felt she could not manage. She was sure his diabetes was out of control and that he was critically ill. He had Cheynes-Stokes respirations, incontinence, and was drinking gallons of water. She did not get any help with the situation until she burst into tears over the telephone and said she absolutely could not handle the situation. The clinic staff were on strike at that time and she was told to take her father to the emergency room. There they confirmed her observations and determined that Mr. X had a blood sugar of 700 (normal is 80–120). He was admitted to the hospital in a confused, weakened state but responded immediately to the administration of insulin, bringing his blood sugar down to 400. His daughter was told that he could go home in 2–3 days. They had a nutritionist teach him about his diet while he was still confused. The daughter said she could not care for him at home, that he was too confused and weak.

Eventually a representative of the HMO helped her explore transfer to a VA hospital. This was accomplished in approximately twelve hours. But her father was not a medical challenge, and his illness was not a service disability, and they wanted him transferred to another facility. The physician turned his case over to a social worker for placement in a nursing home. After two weeks, he was transferred to a VA-approved nursing home, for which the VA would pay for six months.

The daughter had questions about his care at the VA, but felt she had to be careful what she complained about because she didn't want to preclude his returning there if it became necessary. She felt that placing her father in the nursing home was not well thought out or an individualized decision. He was placed on a semi-skilled nursing unit but needed very little care—

primarily food and time orientation. She observed that the people in the various organizations that treated her father—the HMO, the VA (federal system), the nursing home (state system)—did not know what services were available in the other systems. She felt that there was no one to guide them (the patient and family) through the maze from hospital to VA to nursing home.

In the meantime the daughter was taking care of her mother, who was then living alone but did not want to leave her home. The mother was legally blind, suffered from a Parkinsonian-like tremor, and was very weak (weighing less than ninety pounds).

At the end of all this, the daughter was still worrying about whether or not she should try to bring her father home. That was what her mother wanted, but her own energy was depleted and she herself was suffering from tachycardia and osteoarthritis of the spine. Her final remark was "I have to put it all together for myself and my husband and my parents."

In situations like this, patients and their families need someone to relate specifically to them and to assist them as they move in and out of the myriad agencies within the health care system.

Another consumer expressed frustration with the lack of personal care and apparent staff indifference to her situation. She felt that no one knew the answers to her questions or cared to find out. She said she felt "lost in the system." She recommended that consumers be offered clear information about available options, that professionals be more accessible to consumers, that the link between acute and chronic care systems be facilitated and monitored, and that custodial home care be made available at a reasonable cost.

IMPLICATIONS AND RECOMMENDATIONS FOR NURSING PRACTICE

The prospective payment system has ushered in a new world of health care—decreasing use of hospitals and increasing care of patients in the home. The changes have directly affected nursing practice—increasing the emphasis in hospitals on short-term high tech care, increasing the rotation of nursing staff to different units of the hospital and to home care according to census needs, increasing the proportion of nurses working part-time, and increasing the non-nursing tasks performed by nurses. Nursing administrators interviewed in this study were concerned about maintaining an environment in which nurses could function in creative ways; but financial constraints now constitute a "bottom line" issue, particularly in private institutions.

Changes in Hospital Nursing

The inherent nature of the bureaucratic structure of the hospital emphasizes efficiency, predictability, rules, and authority. For at least two decades nursing administrators have tried with varying success to organize nursing practice to facilitate autonomy and creativity within that environment. In the early 60s **team nursing** was introduced. The idea of team nursing was to have a highly qualified nurse responsible for planning the nursing care of a specified group of patients and for supervising a team of associate nurses and nursing aides in implementing this care. The team leader's responsibility was patient care, not unit management as was the case for head nurses. The goal was to develop individualized care plans for patients and to work as an integrated team to carry out those plans. This concept of nursing faded under the pressure of bureaucratic priorities, and the teams reverted to the more segmented, but efficient, function of carrying out assigned tasks.

In order to recapture the personal nature and responsibility of the nurse–patient relationship, which was minimized in the functional approach, **primary nursing** was introduced and received widespread endorsement as a desirable mode of practice. In primary nursing, the designated primary nurse theoretically has twenty-four hour responsibility and accountability for the nursing care of specific patients from hospital admission to discharge. In practice, however, particularly with the present condensed period of hospitalization, primary nursing often falls short of the concept. There may be lag time between patient admission and assignment of the primary nurse. The short period of hospitalization permits little opportunity for the nurse to act on behalf of the patients needs. Primary nurses, in the instances we examined, were expected to carry out routine procedures of patient care on a particular shift and were therefore limited in their freedom to relate to the patient on an ongoing twenty-four hour basis.

The predominate pattern of nursing care in the hospitals studied was **total patient care,** meaning the staff nurse is responsible for the total medical/nursing regimen to be carried out for assigned patients for a particular shift. The focus is on carrying out delegated medical care and assisting patients with activities of daily living. Performance of this role requires judgement in recognizing changes in the patient's condition and in relating the care to a particular patient's situation. The position is subordinate to medicine and permits little autonomy. It is the role of a medical-nursing technician.

Staff nurses have little or no control over when and where they work and minimal participation in decisions affecting patients' care. The part-time, rotating status of the large majority of staff nurses accentuates their lack of control over their work situation and exemplifies the segmented, exchangeable nature of their role in patient care. They are dedicated to high quality care of patients, but financial constraints require that the patient get in and out of the hospital as quickly as possible, and nurses are complying with this objective by streamlining the performance of their tasks. The result is that all staff nurses, regardless of their education or abilities, function primarily as technicians. Head nurses assume some patient care management but are occupied a large part of the time with their unit and personnel management activities. This means that professional nursing is all but lost.

The Need to Differentiate
Professional and Technical Practice

Part of the problem is that there is no clear distinction within the present structure of nursing practice between the roles of the nursing professional and the nursing technician. Both team nursing and primary nursing have specified that the team leader or primary nurse be the "best qualified" nurse and be assisted by "support staff." But in operation these distinctions have not been clear.

Most baccalaureate nursing programs claim that they prepare graduates for entry-level positions in hospitals and other agencies, namely, the staff nurse position. Staff nurses educated at this level, however, are frustrated by their inability to practice what they have learned. Programs of professional education in nursing emphasize the development of critical thinking, decision-making, and independent judgment. Graduates are expected to be able to establish collaborative relationships with a variety of individuals and groups. These characteristics are critically needed in patient care, both within the hospital and the home, but are not fully used in the rapid-paced implementation of medical technology that is characteristic of the staff nurse position. To relieve their frustration, some nurses have sublimated their professional values, others have left hospital nursing for other nursing positions where more autonomy and interpersonal involvement are allowed. Many have given up nursing practice.

The problem is one of a mismatch of education with the expectations of the position. The expectations of the staff nursing position are for a highly skilled technician. Nationally, 66 percent of employed nurses occupy staff positions in hospitals. Interestingly 69 percent of the registered nurses in the United States were educated in either associate degree or diploma programs which are designed to provide technical education. This appears to be a good match between education and expectations of the position.

Differentiation of professional and technical nursing practice is beginning to occur where nurses are employed as patient care coordinators to bridge the gap between hospital and home care. In these situations, the nurse assesses patients' needs for home nursing and families' ability to handle those needs and assists patients with the task of living with various health problems. The nurse serves as a patient advocate and a liaison between patient and other health professionals and agencies. The knowledge base and interpersonal skill needed for these responsibilities are consistent with professional nursing education.

When nursing administrators were asked what they think of a nursing position that permits movement in and out of the hospital according to the patient's needs, they favored the idea but found it hard to envision, possibly because their budgets start and stop at the boundaries of the hospital. Fortunately the restrictions imposed by the boundaries of the old isolated hospital system no longer apply as the new conglomerates in health care delivery encompass hospital and home and beyond. The nurse traditionally the hub of health services within the hospital, or within the home, is becoming an even more effective patient advocate in the new conglomerate.

The Working Environment for Staff Nurses

Continuing to place the burden of non-nursing tasks on the nursing staff is reprehensible. This practice is thought by some administrators to be a way of increasing efficiency but is a source of great dissatisfaction for nurses, a factor which in the long run may not be efficient at all. The expectation that nursing staff will take on additional non-nursing tasks contributes to "working short," a phenomenon associated with low staff cohesiveness, low morale, increased errors, decreased attention to the psychosocial needs of patients, and generally poorer quality and continuity of care.

A major source of dissatisfaction, revealed in this and other studies, is staff nurses' lack of control over their work schedule, particularly the demands that they work weekends and holidays without extra compensation.

In addition, there is no mechanism for recognizing and rewarding outstanding performance at the staff nurse level. There is little external incentive, therefore, to continue performing the physically and emotionally demanding work of a nurse as a life-time career.

Long-Term Care

One of the biggest gaps in the delivery and financing of health care is that there is no organized plan to provide long-term supportive care. The increasing aged population in our society, brings with it an increasing incidence of chronic disease and need for assistance in the activities of daily living. This situation has not been adequately addressed by the current reimbursement system. Home care under Medicare regulations is limited to cases of medical necessity. This rules out the assistance needed for patients with a variety of degenerative diseases. It does not provide for continuing care on a long-term basis either in a nursing home or at home. Patients and families who need long-term nursing care do not know how to obtain it, and even if they can find it, there is little financial assistance for this kind of care. A master plan for the coordination and financing of acute and long-term care is desperately needed now and will become increasingly imperative.

Matching Responsibility and Authority for Patient Care

The present system of reimbursement for health care services is riddled with confusion about the authority for determining needed patient care. Medicare regulations specify that home nursing care must be authorized by a physician on the basis of medical necessity rather than by a nurse on the basis of nursing care needs. In practice, the nurse doing the discharge planning usually assesses the patient's needs for home nursing and then obtains the physician's approval of this plan. On the other hand, nurses are being employed by HMOs as utilization reviewers and given the authority to make decisions regarding eligibility for treatment based on medical need. In practice, physicians develop the guidelines for determining appropriate medical care, and nurses follow these guidelines in making decisions affecting other physicians' practice. These situations set up a continuing adversarial relationship between physicians and nurses rather than promoting a collaboration that would yield the best possible care for patients. It seems reasonable that physicians monitor medical care and nurses monitor nursing care, and that the goal be the integration of the two.

CONCLUSION

Within the context of the present prospective payment system the role of the hospital staff nurse is that of a medical–nursing technician and is most appropriately performed by RNs educated in programs emphasizing technical education. Even though the total number of nursing positions has decreased along with reductions in hospital occupancy, there will be an increased need for highly skilled technicians in critical care. The continuing expansion of home nursing care will be accompanied by an increased need for RNs skilled in technical care in the home.

Patients and their families have a critical need for nurses who serve as patient care coordinators and are accessible on a continuing basis prior to, during, and following acute care episodes. Such nurses should have a professional nursing education. The responsibilities of this position include assessment and authorization of a patient's need for nursing care and coordination of the services of associate nurses in implementing that care. By serving as patient advocates and liaisons with other health professionals and agencies, these nurses can assure continuity and quality of care.

CHAPTER EIGHTEEN

Toward an Integrative Model of Professional Practice

Margaret A. Newman

The "so-called" nursing shortage is not a shortage in the usual sense . . . the problem is one of . . . failure to implement recommendations . . . [which] propose action relating to environment of practice . . . ; the restructuring of practice itself; the preparation of nurses and changes needed in the profession . . .

Myrtle K. Aydelotte
Testimony to Secretary's Commission on Nursing,
Department of Health and Human Services
March 7, 1988

THE NURSING PROFESSION has been slow to transform the theory and practice of nursing into a professional model. The nature of professional education remains an unresolved issue that is paralleled by lack of delineation of professional practice. Models of practice have come and gone with seemingly equivocal results. Theory development and research, though having received considerable attention over the past decade, have had a questionable impact on practice. These essential aspects of the profession have developed, for the most part,

Reprinted with permission from *Journal of Professional Nursing,* 6(3): 167–173, 1990. Copyright © 1990 by W. B. Saunders Company.

along separate paths, and the lack of communication among nursing educators, practitioners, and scientists has become untenable. The urgency brought about by the nursing shortage and the decrease in applicants to nursing educational programs has exposed the lack of a clear professional model and prompted a collaborative effort to remedy the situation. The recent attention to case management models of practice offers a needed dimension to professional practice; yet the coordination of nursing case management with the existing models of practice remains unarticulated, and the education required for different levels of practice has not been made explicit.

The lack of specificity of level of education for practice roles is a major problem with current models of practice. A prevailing theme of a recent invitational conference on the future of nursing at the University of Pennsylvania, Philadelphia, PA, was the concern of participants regarding the lack of differentiation of practice roles according to educational preparation (Fagin, 1987). Altman (1987) portrayed the problem graphically by pointing out that "squishing" together all RNs or "lumping" baccalaureate graduates in with graduates of other programs "destroys" baccalaureate nursing. Mechanic (1987) decried the lack of differentiated structure over the "whole arena" of nursing. *Three decades ago* Rogers (1961) proposed a model of differentiated practice according to educational preparation, stating "refusal to state frankly a clear differentiation of levels of nursing constitutes one of the most significant problems facing nurses *today* (emphasis added)." The time is long overdue for the profession to move from having nurses with various levels of preparation doing the same thing, or nurses with one level of preparation doing everything, to practitioners with different levels of preparation doing different, interrelated things.

Primm's (1987) model of differentiation of practice of the baccalaureate nurse from the associate degree nurse represents a step toward clarifying this dilemma and several demonstrations of differentiated practice are underway. This model differentiates the baccalaureate nurse from the associate degree nurse in terms of complexity of care provided, range of clients served, structure of the environment in which practice occurs, and level of communication and organizational skills.

The task of differentiation is not complete, however, without differentiation of the competencies of the nurse prepared at the graduate level and specification of how this nurse articulates with nurses in the other two categories.

DEVELOPMENT OF THE NURSING PROFESSION

A brief overview of the sequential development of nursing models of practice, in relation to educational programs and knowledge base, portends the need for integration of the beliefs, knowledges, and practices in an overall structure of professional practice.

The progression of models of nursing practice over the years has followed growth cycles suggested by Ainsworth-Land (1982; Land, 1973). The first stage is referred to as *formative,* a stage in which the phenomenon (in this case, nursing) is in the process of becoming itself and establishing its identity. The change that takes place is accretive: it expands and becomes more of itself.

In the formative stage, when nursing was in the process of becoming itself and establishing its identity, the persons who performed nursing duties were primarily women who were family members or neighbors. They cared for persons who were sick and in need of nurturing on a one-to-one basis, usually in the home (Reverby, 1987). They learned from each other in an informal apprenticeship, passing on knowledge gained through intuition and the process of trial and error. They were in control of and responsible for their services.

The second stage of development, according to Ainsworth-Land, is characterized as *normative,* a stage in which the phenomenon in interaction with the environment loses some of the authority and expansion of the first stage, becomes embroiled in hierarchical structures, and develops a competitive, persuasive stance in trying to establish and maintain its own territory.

The beginning development of medical technology with its emphasis on hospital care set the stage for the changes that took place in nursing's second stage of development. Nurses relinquished their independent status and became employees of hospitals and subordinates to physicians (Ashley, 1976). The tasks of hospital management and medical technology began to usurp the time and energy of nurses, and nursing services to clients became fragmented. The early formal apprenticeship education was controlled by hospitals.

The knowledge base during this period was determined predominantly by the medical paradigm. Basic values of personalized care remained central to nursing's professed calling, but they provided little direction for the formal development of nursing's knowledge (Newman, 1972).

In the third stage, *integrative,* the system begins to relate to other systems in the environment in a cooperative, mutual way. A partnership approach becomes the predominant way of life. Ainsworth-Land (1982) suggests that as a system moves into a new stage of development, it incorporates the best from previous stages. Such a process would involve the synthesis of the individualized intuitive caring of stage I with the medical knowledge and management skills of stage II into a nursing paradigm that integrates caring, medical technology, and organizational skill in a completely new view of health and health care. The knowledge base for nursing practice during the long period between early solo practice and relatively recent independent practice has been dominated by the medical paradigm, but as nurses have become aware of a distinctly nursing perspective, they have explicated the philosophical and theoretical foundations of nursing, and there is now some agreement on the nursing paradigm that forms the foundation for practice (Roy, 1984; Sarter, 1988).

Table 18.1 depicts the characteristics of nursing in stages I and II and suggests characteristics of integration in stage III. Temporal demarcation between stages of development is not absolute.

Table 18.1 Characteristics of the Development of the Nursing Profession According to Ainsworth-Land's Stages of Growth

	Stage I: Formative	Stage II: Normative	Stage III: Integrative
Education	Informal apprenticeship	Formalized apprenticeship Controlled by service agency Organized by medical paradigm	Professional model University based Organized by nursing paradigm
Practice	Solo provider in the home One-to-one relationship Comfort measures and assistance with activities of daily living	Setting-specific employees of hospitals or community Subordinates to physicians Functional care to multiple clients and/or "total" care combining medical treatments and assistance with activities of daily living Hospital management	Individual care integrating one-to-one with team approach Transformation of technology into person-centered transformative caring Collaborative relationship with clients and other health professionals
Knowledge	Intuitive caring Based on experience	Medical paradigm/technology Nursing pre-paradigm	Nursing paradigm

MOVEMENT TOWARD AN
INTEGRATIVE STAGE

Efforts to implement new practice models over the past 25 years illustrate movement in the direction of an integrative stage. One of the first attempts to transform nursing into a cooperative endeavor was the introduction of *team nursing*. During the 1940s and 1950s there was a proliferation of educational programs preparing different levels of practitioners in nursing, as well as a gradual increase in baccalaureate education in nursing. Team nursing was introduced in the early 1960s as a way of using practitioners with various levels of education in a coordinated way to provide planned, individualized care to clients under the leadership of a baccalaureate nurse. The key to team nursing was the conceptualization of a different role for the team leader, who was charged with the responsibility for the nature and quality of care administered by the team and for determining the appropriate match of clients' needs with the qualifications of the team members. The team concept had the potential for combining different levels of personnel in creative ways, but was never implemented fully, perhaps because the professional role of the team leader was not fully understood and was not reserved solely for the baccalaureate graduate. In addition each team was time-bound by shift work; so the leadership (and possibly the plan of care) varied from shift to shift. This brief attempt to implement a team approach to individualized care faded, and the organization of patient care tended to revert to the previous functional, segmented method.

By the early 1970s, in another attempt to recapture the personal nature and responsibility of a one-to-one nurse-patient relationship, *primary nursing* became the predominant model of care. The need for continuity of care across shifts was addressed by designating a primary nurse as responsible for the planning and implementation of nursing care for a particular patient for the entire period of hospitalization. The intent was that the primary nurse had 24-hour responsibility for the patient's care, participated in the care as necessary to gain a full understanding of the patient's situation, and determined what nursing care the patient was to receive. When the primary nurse was not assuming the direct care, other nurses and auxiliary personnel were expected to follow the primary nurse's directions for care (Manthey, 1980).

While there is a general perception that primary nursing models were a positive innovation, few studies clearly support beneficial outcomes (Giovanetti, 1985). Part of the difficulty may have been the lack of consistency in the operationalization of primary nursing. When used in acute care institutions, the primary nurse typically has been required to work a shift as well as fulfill the primary nurse role; the form the care has taken more accurately resembles what has been referred to as "total patient care," which was assumed by another nurse when the primary nurse was not on duty (Newman & Autio, 1986). Lack of control over their time has constituted a major frustration for nurses (Aiken, 1987). In order to fulfill their responsibilities, primary nurses often worked beyond their designated shift without compensation (Rabkin, 1987; Goertzen, 1987). Even so, with the advent of shortened periods of hospitalization, a client could undergo a period of hospitalization without ever seeing a primary nurse (Newman & Autio, 1986). Primary nurses, therefore, have not been free to organize their work to span the 24-hour period. The primary nursing model was based on teamwork around the clock, but it did not provide a structure that would enable the primary nurse to exercise continuing responsibility. Educators have indicated that a baccalaureate was needed for the primary nurse, but in practice the preparation for primary nursing has not been explicit and has varied considerably (Manthey, 1980; Fagin & Goodwin, 1972).

The current rapid movement of clients in and out of hospitals and the need for supportive services in the home has accentuated the need for coordination of nursing services across settings (Newman & Autio, 1986; Rusch, 1986). In that respect the *case manager* model of practice has moved the profession a step closer to a professional model. Case management has been defined as a systematic process of health assessment, planning, intervention, service coordination and/or referral, and monitoring through which the multiple-service needs of clients are met (American Nurses' Association, 1988; Ethridge & Lamb, 1989; Parker & Secord, 1988). Evaluation of the implementation of nursing case management shows not only significant increases in patient satisfaction and nursing job satisfaction but also savings in the cost of health services (Ethridge & Lamb, 1989; Wolf et al., 1985/1986; Zander et al., 1988).

But like its predecessors, the case manager model presents itself in various forms. Ideally, nurse case managers are responsible and accountable for the overall plan of *nursing* care of clients on a continuing basis across a broad spectrum of care settings: in the hospital, the home, and other community health care centers. This model of case management is being practiced in some instances (Ethridge & Rusch, 1989). In others, however, the responsibilities of the case manager are limited primarily to the immediate period surrounding hospitalization (Koerner et al., 1988; Zander, 1988). In the latter instance the focus of the practice is related primarily to management of *medical* care in an expeditious manner.

In other instances, though not labeled as such, clinical nurse specialists have functioned as effective case managers (Brooten et al., 1986). Public health nurses traditionally have functioned as case managers for a circumscribed population in the community setting and continue to do so (American Nurses' Association, 1988). Nurse practitioners, too, often function in roles congruent with the case management concept in a variety of settings. Evaluation of their practice indicates that they improve access to health care services and continuity of care by matching the needs of patients with appropriate services and by coordinating the care of many health professionals (U.S. Congress, 1986). Still needed is a structure for articulating the role of clinical nurse specialists and nurse practitioners with the larger arena of nursing practice.

Variation in the implementation of the case manager model lies, also, in the level of educational preparation required of the case manager. In some instances, registered nurses, regardless of their level of preparation, have been used as case managers; in others the case managers must have a minimum of a baccalaureate. A number of case managers have master's or higher degrees (Rusch, 1988), and there is some consensus that graduate preparation is needed for the knowledge base and decision-making skill required of the case manager (Cronen & Maklebust, 1989; Stull, 1987).

A PROPOSED TRILEVEL MODEL OF PRACTICE

The development of nursing practice has paralleled the growing complexity of the health care delivery system and now requires the integration of at least three different practice roles in order for the professional model to be complete.

First, there is a need for a professional nursing clinician with direct responsibility to clients over time for the determination of both short- and long-term nursing care across multiple practice settings including home care. This role incorporates characteristics of roles variously labeled case manager, patient care coordinator, clinical nurse specialist, and nurse practitioner. Professional practice involves a direct connection between the professional and the client for an identifiable service in a particular area of expertise. It is not bound by place or time. In order for a professional relationship to be satisfying to both the professional and the client, it must evolve over time (Thorne & Robinson, 1988). Educational preparation needed for this role is a post-baccalaureate professional degree based on a curriculum that is person-centered and focused on health, as opposed to setting-specific and organized by medical specialties. Case management connotes the mode of practice; clinical specialization connotes the area of expertise. The chosen area of specialization may be as general as long-term care of the elderly or as specific as midwifery.

Second, there is a need for a nurse who provides clinical leadership within institutional settings or service agencies (here called team leader) and is responsible around the clock for the quality of nursing care administered by a team of staff nurses and auxiliary personnel. This role combines aspects of the roles previously ascribed to team leader and primary nurse but without the limitations of shift work expectations. Preparation needed for this role is a baccalaureate in nursing.

Third, there is a continuing need for staff nurses who are responsible for the implementation of delegated medical and nursing care for designated clients within a specified setting and who function as members of a nursing team. Preparation needed for this role is the associate degree in nursing. (Until transition to associate degree education is complete, it is reasonable to expect nurses prepared in diploma and practical nursing programs to fill some staff positions.) A comparison of the educational preparation, structure of practice, and role responsibilities of the three roles is shown in Table 18.2. An elaboration of the differentiation of the curricula of the three programs is beyond the purpose of this article, but it would correspond to the responsibilities designated for each practice role.

This trilevel model declares all three roles to be essential to the implementation of nursing's practice responsibilities. The nursing clinician relates directly to clients throughout the period of their need for nursing consultation and service wherever the need for care arises and maintains a collegial relationship with other health professionals involved in the client's care. The responsibilities of this nurse are for collaboration with the client for total health assessment and long-term planning. These responsibilities are coordinated with those of the nursing team leader and staff nurses in hospitals, home care, and other health care settings. The fulfillment of the clinician role provides clients with direct and individualized access to a single professional nurse on an ongoing basis regardless of the setting in which care occurs.

Table 18.2 Educational Preparation, Structure of Practice, and Role Responsibilities of a Trilevel Model of Professional Practice

	Clinician	Team Leader	Staff Nurse
Educational preparation	Postbaccalaureate	Baccalaureate	Associate degree
Structure of practice	Direct long-term relationship with clients for determination and coordination of nursing care across multiple settings	Continuous responsibility for clinical leadership of nursing staff in specific, structured care context, e.g., institutional settings or service agencies	Time- and place-limited responsibility for delegated care of assigned clients
Role responsibilities	Primary relationship with client for the purpose of identifying health care needs and facilitating clients' decision making regarding action to be taken	Transformation and interpretation of prescribed medical and nursing care according to individualized, client-centered needs	Implementation of delegated medical and nursing care for specific clients according to plans developed by nursing clinician and team leader
	Communication and collaboration with nurses in various settings where client is being cared for regarding relationship of immediate care to long-term perspective	Matching of client's needs with staff abilities	Communication of observations regarding client's condition and effectiveness of care
	Collaboration with other health professionals to facilitate client's access to needed resources	Integration of nursing care within interdisciplinary context	

The baccalaureate nurse is designated as team leader within specific, circumscribed care settings including home care. The team leader's critical contribution to care is in the translation of medical technology into individualized, personalized care and in the coordination of the immediate nursing care of clients in the hospital, home, or other care agency with the overall, long-term nursing plan as determined mutually by the nursing clinician and client. The team leader plays an important role in maximizing the contributions of nursing team members by matching their abilities with the individual needs of clients for care.

The staff nurse is responsible for implementing the delegated nursing-medical care. This role is not unlike the current staff nurse role except that it is more thoroughly integrated into professional nursing practice by the team relationships and decisions. A schematic representation of the three nursing roles, their relationships to clients, and their position in the health care system is provided in Figure 18.1. Each of the roles is distinctively different, yet interdependent. Each requires different educational preparation; each is essential to the whole of professional practice. The nursing clinician functions directly with

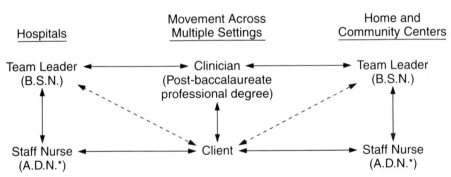

*Includes diploma graduate and L.P.N. through transition to associate degree education.

Figure 18.1 Diagram of Relationship of Practitioners in a Trilevel Model.

clients on an ongoing basis in different settings. The team leader functions in one setting, but spans the 24-hour daily care period in order to maintain ongoing responsibility for the quality of nursing care of clients assigned to the team and provide leadership for staff. The staff nurse's activity is limited to specific care assignments within a specific space-time structure.

FURTHER CONSIDERATIONS

Implementation of the proposed model will require a hospital infrastructure that supports professional practice in nursing. As is evident in stage II, nurses traditionally have taken on responsibility for management of the entire delivery system, not just nursing care. This tendency has expanded with decentralization of administrative tasks and responsibilities. It is the assumption of this model that in order for nurses to be free to fulfill their professional care responsibilities to clients, hospital administration will need to assume unit management responsibilities and provide auxiliary staff to perform non-nursing tasks. A recent survey by the Hay Group, a management consulting firm in Philadelphia, PA, demonstrated that 52 percent of nurses' time was consumed by nonprofessional tasks, a factor that has been implicated in nursing job dissatisfaction and burnout (Misuse of RNs, 1989; Schere, 1987). The interface of the proposed model of practice with hospital management and other health professional practice will require further consideration and careful working out of collegial relationships. Progress thus far indicates that nurse case managers are establishing themselves as a pivotal point in the delivery of health care (Rusch, 1988).

The responsibility of the professional practitioner in nursing is primarily to the client and secondarily to interdisciplinary cooperation and to organizational needs of the system. The differentiation and integration of three different practice roles based on three levels of education provides a structure for the whole of nursing's professional practice commitment. The cooperation inherent in the articulation of the three roles will decrease the competition between different levels of practitioners. The internal coordination of nursing practice that is the potential of this model will make it possible to interact with the larger system of health care in a coordinated way and thereby send a clear message regarding the contribution that nursing is making to health care.

A final word: At a recent National League for Nursing convention, Carolyne Davis warned, "The time-frame is short to restore clinical time for nurses, remodel the workplace, and restructure education to produce a more advanced clinical competency base" (Davis, 1989). *The time is now.*

REFERENCES

Aiken, L. (1987). Nurses for the future: Breaking the shortage cycles. *American Journal of Nursing, 87*, 1616–1620.

Ainsworth-Land, G., & V. (1982). *Forward to basics.* Buffalo, NY: DOK.

Altman, S. (1987). Nurses for the future: What does a BS degree buy? (Discussion) *American Journal of Nursing, 87*, 1630.

American Nurses' Association. (1988). *Nursing case management.* Kansas City, MO: American Nurses' Association.

Ashley, J. A. (1976). *Hospitals, paternalism, and the role of the nurse.* New York: Teachers College Press.

Brooten, D., Kumar, S., Brown, L. P., et al. (1986). A randomized clinical trial of early hospital discharge and home follow-up care of very-low-birth-weight infants. *New England Journal of Medicine, 315*, 934–939.

Cronin, C. J., & Maklebust, J. (1989). Case-managed care: Capitalizing on the CNS. *Nursing Management, 20,* 38–47.

Davis, C. (1989). "Time is short" to restructure RNs' education. *American Journal of Nursing, 89,* 1083.

Ethridge, P., & Lamb, G. S. (1989). Professional nursing case management improves quality, access and costs. *Nursing Management, 20,* 30–35.

Ethridge, P., & Rusch, S. C. (1989). Professional nurse/case manager in changing organizational structures. In M. Johnson (Ed.), *Changing organizational structures. Iowa nursing administration series* (Vol. 2, pp. 146–164). Redwood City, CA: Addison-Wesley.

Fagin, C. M. (1987). Nurses for the future. *American Journal of Nursing, 87,* 1593–1648.

Fagin, C. M., & Goodwin, B. (1972). Baccalaureate preparation for primary care. *Nursing Outlook, 20,* 240–244.

Giovanetti, P. (1985). Evaluation of nursing research. In H. H. Werley & J. J. Fitzpatrick (Eds.), *Annual review of nursing research* (Vol. 4, pp. 127–151). New York: Springer.

Goertzen, I. (1987). Nurses for the future: What does a BS degree buy? (Discussion) *American Journal of Nursing, 87,* 1629.

Koerner, J. G., Bunkers, L. B., Nelson, B., et al. (1988). *Implementing differentiated practice: The Sioux Valley Hospital experience.* Unpublished manuscript.

Land, G. T. L. (1973). *Grow or die.* New York: Dell.

Manthey, M. (Ed.). (1980). *The practice of primary nursing.* Boston, MA: Blackwell Scientific.

Mechanic, D. (1987). Nurses for the future: What does a BS degree buy? (Discussion) *American Journal of Nursing, 87,* 1630.

Misuse of RNs spurs shortage, says new study "Only 26% of time is spent in professional care." (1989). *American Journal of Nursing, 89,* 1223+.

Newman, M. A. (1972). Nursing's theoretical evolution. *Nursing Outlook, 34,* 359–366.

Newman, M. A., & Autio, S. (1986). *Nursing in a prospective payment system health care environment.* Minneapolis: University of Minnesota School of Nursing.

Parker, M., & Secord, L. J. (1988). Case managers: Guiding the elderly through the health care maze. *American Journal of Nursing, 88,* 1674–1676.

Primm, P. L. (1987). Differentiated practice for ADN- and BSN-prepared nurses. *Journal of Professional Nursing, 3,* 218–224.

Rabkin, M. (1987). Nurses for the future: What does a BS degree buy? (Discussion) *American Journal of Nursing, 87,* 1628–1629.

Reverby, S. (1987). A caring dilemma: Womanhood and nursing in historical perspective. *Nursing Research, 36,* 5–11.

Rogers, M. E. (1961). *Educational revolution in nursing.* New York: Macmillan.

Roy, C. (1984). Framework for classification systems development progress and issues. In M. J. Kim, G. K. McFarland, & A. M. McLane (Eds.), *Classification of nursing diagnoses proceedings of the fifth national conference* (pp. 26–40). St. Louis, MO: Mosby.

Rusch, S. C. (1986). Continuity of care: From hospital unit into home. *Nursing Management, 17,* 38–41.

Rusch, S. C. (1988). Case management model. Paper presented at "Shaping the future of nursing: Minnesota's vision." St. Paul, MN, September 9–10.

Sarter, B. (1988). Philosophical sources of nursing theory. *Nursing Science Quarterly, 1,* 52–59.

Schere, P. (1987). When every day is Saturday: The shortage. *American Journal of Nursing, 87,* 1284–1290.

Stull, M. K. (1987). Entry to practice roundtable. *Current Concepts in Nursing, 1,* 2–12.

Thorne, S. E., & Robinson, C. A. (1988). Health care relationships: The chronic illness perspective. *Research in Nursing and Health, 11,* 293–300.

U.S. Congress, Office of Technology Assessment. (1986). *Nurse practitioners, physician assistants, and certified nurse midwives: A policy analysis* (Health Care Technology Study 37). Washington, DC: U.S. Government Printing Office.

Wolf, R. S., Halas, K. T., Green, L. B., et al. (1985/1986). A model for the integration of community-based health and social services. *Home Health Care Services Quarterly, 6,* 41–57.

Zander, K. (1988). Nursing case management: Strategic management of cost and quality outcomes. *Journal of Nursing Administration, 18,* 23–30.

Zander, K., Blaney, C., Hayes, J., et al. (1988). Nursing group practice: "The Cadillac" in continuity. *Definition: The Center for Nursing Case Management, 3*(2)1–2. (Newsletter, Department of Nursing, New England Medical Center, Boston, MA).

CHAPTER NINETEEN

Nurse Case Management: The Coming Together of Theory and Practice

Margaret A. Newman

Gerri S. Lamb

Cathy Michaels

CARONDELET ST. MARY'S Hospital and Health Center, Tucson, Arizona, has become a national center for demonstration and exchange of ideas regarding nursing case management. This article represents and incorporates a dialogue among the authors and the nurse case managers and their clients at St. Mary's regarding the philosophy and theory underlying their nursing practice.

SETTING THE STAGE FOR DIALOGUE

Newman: I first had the opportunity to meet with the nurse case managers at St. Mary's in October 1988, at which time we had a mutual exchange in terms of their practice and my theory. This exchange piqued my interest in exploring the nature of their practice in a more systematic way. In December 1989, I returned to spend 3 months interacting with the nurse case managers at St. Mary's, attending their group meetings, participating in home visits, and mainly just talking to them about their practice. The primary purpose of my visit was to describe the nature of nursing case management at St. Mary's and the interrelationships of nursing case management with the larger nursing and health care community. I was also interested in evaluating the relevance of my theory of health and nursing to their practice, but considered that a secondary objective, to be addressed after I had accomplished the first.

Lamb and Michaels: Prior to Margaret's initial visit to St. Mary's, the nurse case managers group had talked with each other at some length about our practice. We had explored what some felt were the central elements of our work with clients and ways we were able to assist clients. The intent of our many exchanges, both formal and informal, was to share views about our work and to learn from one another. During these meetings it was common to hear phrases like "facilitating choice" and "respect for where the client is at." When we first met with Margaret in October 1988, we spent our brief time together telling her about our practice as nurse case managers. In turn, she described and diagrammed her theory. For many of the nurse case managers present at the initial meeting, there was a sense that Margaret's theory could provide a new way of looking at and understanding our practice. We were eager to explore our work from the perspective of a nursing theory. Our goals for Margaret's 3-month stay were to gain new insights about our practice and to examine the relevance of her theory to our reality of nurse case management. We hoped this experience would help us translate the process and outcomes of our practice in a more communicable manner.

Newman: As I began my study of nurse case management at St. Mary's, I searched for a form of cooperative inquiry that would permit full participation of all involved parties, including myself. A hermeneutic dialectic process provided a guide for initiating and conducting interviews with the nurse case managers, nursing administrators, and selected hospital nursing staff (Guba & Lincoln, 1989). This process involved a continuing dialectic of iteration, analysis, reiteration, and reanalysis, leading to the emergence of a joint construction of the experience. I began the interviews of the nurse case managers with very general questions, such as, "What is the most meaningful part of your role as a case manager?" and "How do you relate to other nurses in the system?" The meaning and structure of the situation began to take form through my analysis of the data. In addition to the open-ended unstructured questions, my analysis was shared with the next respondents, and their response in turn was incorporated in the developing structure. I was free also to offer my response to the shared information; my point of view entered into these dialogues but was not the major focus, which was on their experiences in case management. I talked individually with 14 case managers and 6 hospital nursing administrators or staff and participated in both formal and informal case manager group meetings. At the close of the 3 months, I shared my synthesis of the data and its relevance to my theory with the case manager group.

BACKGROUND OF NURSE CASE MANAGEMENT AT ST. MARY'S

In 1985, recognizing the increasing need for extending nursing services beyond the hospital and beyond what Medicare and other third-party payors would support at that time, Phyllis Ethridge, vice president for Patient Care Services, initiated a nurse case management (NCM) program at St. Mary's. Her intent was to offer direct nursing services to vulnerable and high-risk individuals across hospital and community settings. The program began with one nurse case manager (NCMr) functioning out of the inpatient pulmonary unit and, at the time of this study, had grown to 18 NCMrs with diverse clinical backgrounds and areas of expertise. New members joined the program as the number of clientele increased, a factor related both to the increasing recognition of high-risk health concerns of clients and also to the emergence of new health care purchasers seeking contracts with NCM.

PHILOSOPHICAL AND PROFESSIONAL ORIENTATION

The philosophical underpinnings of the NCM practice are important: The emphasis is on the whole, truly looking at the whole. Several of the NCMrs attributed their views and personal growth to traditional Indian medicine, a holistic philosophy that closely ties the spiritual dimension of a person and the environment with all other aspects. Others expressed an equally holistic perspective emanating from their own personal beliefs and experiences. Caring and a commitment to service are inherent in their purpose.

The title *case manager* does not reflect the holistic framework that is the foundation for practice at St. Mary's. The NCMr does not attempt to control or manage the client's situation. On the contrary, the NCMr works to build the patient's self-reliance by respecting her or his decisions and facilitating informed choices. Some of the NCMrs, having come from the controlled environment of hospital care, have found it necessary to let go of their own professional and personal agendas in order to be fully present with the client, that is, to attend to the *client's* agenda: what is important to them, what choices they are faced with, and how the unfolding of those choices will take place.

The use of the NCMr title reflects the emphasis placed on cost-effectiveness as well as quality. When cost containment became a force within the health care delivery system, case management regained a following. It was a role that enabled health professionals to match individual need with services and settings in such a way that cost-effectiveness and quality were both enhanced. Although other health professionals serve as case managers, nurses are able to offer a more comprehensive assessment of health by combining case management with direct nursing care. Through pattern recognition, NCMrs engage the clients in viewing and managing their health in creative ways that enable clients to seek medical and hospital services at a lower severity of illness, thereby incurring a less costly and less dramatic illness episode. Moreover with earlier pattern recognition, clients are enabled to seek health alternatives, not just episodic illness services.

Case management as practiced at St. Mary's is simply a vehicle for practicing professional nursing. It exemplifies the essence of nursing that was always there but was overshadowed at times by response to external demands. The NCMrs are known to their clients simply as nurses. NCM is similar to community health nursing, but is more fully integrated with the total spectrum of acute-to-chronic phases of care. NCMrs are not bound by space or time; they establish ongoing partnerships with people and move across the spectrum of health care settings. They are organizationally empowered to carry out professional service, providing direct care, as well as brokering resources and services. Referral of clients to the NCMr most often occurs at the time of hospital discharge but may come at any time that clients are perceived as needing assistance with their or their family's needs in managing health concerns. Referrals are made by the hospital nursing staff, social service, physicians, and other clients.

The NCMrs function in a non-hierarchical model of group practice. The work of the group is defined by the group and carried out by each member. While each NCMr maintains responsibility for his or her practice, decisions involving the whole group, for example, regarding new contracts or on-call system, are brought to the group. Decisions are made by building consensus, and each group member has an equal opportunity to participate in decision making.

The focus of each individual's practice is determined in different ways. Some NCMrs serve clients linked to particular units within the hospital and others serve clients associated with an established health care program or funding agency. Each person has a loosely designated area of practice reflective of individual expertise, for example, low-income maternal-child health, problems of the frail elderly, Native American health problems, families with long-term care problems such as diabetes and Alzheimer's disease, or families facing decisions regarding withdrawal of nutrition and treatment from comatose patients.

DIMENSIONS OF THE
PROFESSIONAL RELATIONSHIP

The most important thing about NCM is the *relationship* formed with the client. It may be short-term or long-term. It is characterized by compassion, continuity, and respect for the client's choice. The focus is on process: the process of the client-environment interaction and the process of the nurse-client relationship.

Pattern recognition. Seeing clients in the home in relation to their families over time facilitates recognition of the whole. One NCMr said that when she worked in the hospital, illness was seen as an episode, but in her work as a NCMr, it is seen as a way of life. For example, one client, a fiercely independent 75-year-old woman who lived alone, was receiving chemotherapy monthly for treatment of lymphoma. Before and immediately following chemotherapy, she was often weak and unable to prepare her food or do more than a sponge bath. Although money was not an issue for her, she had chosen not to hire someone to assist her with her personal care. She believed that paid help would not only provide personal care but also would make decisions for her and in essence take over her life. She seemed to express her aliveness most when confronting the challenge of performing activities of daily living and home management. At this time in her life, when her body was accelerating its physical decline, the pattern of her life may be characterized as struggling to maintain control.

Another NCMr said that it is not necessary, or perhaps not possible, to understand the whole (pattern) of the process but just to recognize it and accept it: "What I'm doing is dealing with someone else's process. I may not understand. I just recognize it and offer them choices. They're *expanding their process,* and that's how they choose to do it" (italics added).

The ability to acknowledge and facilitate the expression of the client's pattern distinguishes the professional expertise of the NCMr from the ministrations of a concerned friend. When pattern recognition occurs, clients sense that the NCMr "knows me" and is able to assist in bringing about desired changes in their lives.

Rhythm and timing. . . . The nurse-client relationship is rhythmic, and timing is important: when to connect and when to separate. One NCMr said, "It's hard to anticipate the 'success' of the relationship. Sometimes right timing takes place. They call you at the right time. . . . That [incident of helping a client] was just one little intervention that she was ready for. I saw that as being important."

And another saw the practice "as a rhythmic, dynamic process of opening to self, to others, to alternate ways of living health. Timing is important. Knowing (sensing) when 'this is enough.'" The NCMr continued:

> This is illustrated in my relationship with N.E., a 74-year-old woman, who is diabetic, legally blind and an amputee of 50 years. She has been wheelchair-bound since she fractured her good leg one year ago. She often feels overwhelmed by her body's physical decline and the accompanying social isolation. When she has been ready to express her feelings of confinement and explore options for opening her world, I made weekly home visits. When she returned to insulin use, I made weekly home visits plus three to four telephone calls per week for about one and a half months. During times when N.E. lets me know in her ways that it is not her time for change, I allowed the interval between visits to increase to a month and relied on her to call me if needed.

In NCM practice, both the client and the nurse are relatively autonomous and relate to each other in a rhythmic process. The NCMrs have become aware of the timing and rhythm of working with their clients. Freed from usual bureaucratic time constraints, the NCMr and client can orchestrate their interactions to match optimal times for growth and change. NCMrs can move in and out of the client's environment according to client needs, client readiness, and the NCMr's ability and comfort in the situation.

Opening of self. The opening of self to the client is at the heart of the relationship, as described by two of the NCMRs:

> That to me is what my practice is all about: to be open, continue feeling and learning and be prepared for the questions that come up and be prepared to sense where the clients are and what it is they're really asking for and be able to work it in every aspect of their being . . .

> •

> It's hard to say that being there is doing something, but it is. . . . The task is to stay filled and remain open—it has to do with letting go; less is more sometimes.

One nurse pointed out that she is able to utilize herself totally, the whole of herself, in the process: "I bring everything I can (who I am, my experiences, the fact that I'm a mother) to the process—it's not only okay, it's important!"

The opening of self to the rhythm and timing of the relationship is a crucial dimension of authenticity in the nurse-client relationship.

Mutual growth. The process experienced by the NCMrs is one of mutual growth:

> I wish I could describe what this job has done for me as a person because that almost blows my mind more than what has happened with clients.

> •

[Previous academic] learning became relevant in this environment—the demand for integration—I look at things differently!

And the practice expands as the NCMr expands:

It was a personal and professional stretch to look at the whole, to deal with areas I hadn't dealt with before . . . as one grows professionally and personally, new options open up. I'm sharing my experience with the person [client], [just] as what they're going through is offered to me. I hear things and recognize things in people that I wouldn't have before, might have dealt with differently.

Another NCMr tells of the mutual unfolding process that takes place in the nurse-client relationship:

In the beginning of our partnership, P.H., a 72-year-old woman with multiple health problems, was distrustful of strangers. In the year and a half we have been working together, P.H. is learning to be more trusting, voices responsibility for her ailment, and laughs more. In general, she enjoys more lighter days. I, in turn, have learned to dance more sensitively in her presence. If I come to her home visit with her health assessment checklist in mind, she is quiet and answers only in monosyllables. If, instead, I follow the unfolding process, she initiates conversations and shares her concerns and issues. I have learned there is no shorthanding our process, even when she is trusting of me.

Choices. Several of the NCMrs characterized their work as having respect for clients' choices and facilitating their choices. The subtleties of the NCMr's role in this process have not been fully explored, but one NCMr felt the word *facilitate* implied more direction in the process than she was comfortable with; she saw the relationship as one of "allowing" the client to choose. Another NCMr pointed out the obstructive nature of labeling and inflexible judgment in the process: "Judgment about a situation, say 'She's hopeless,' cuts it off—there's nothing more to do. It is very efficient. No one is ever going to make you fill out an incident report for not getting to the point of what's going on, but they will if you don't do this or that."

A particular concern was how to support clients' choices in an unconditional, nonjudgmental way, especially when the choices oppose the medical plan of care or are contrary to one's own values: "You have to meet them where they are. A judgment cuts off [possibilities]. It's not okay to reject them [clients] when they say things contrary to [one's own beliefs]."

Here are some of the choices faced by the clients and the NCMrs:

- Choices made by the wife of a man with Alzheimer's disease: recognizing the disease and the limitations it imposes, refusing further treatment, accepting respite care, taking care of herself, putting her husband in a care facility.

- The nurse's dilemma of how to accept and support a young mother's behavioral choice not to care for her baby.

- The nurse's choice of how to support a client's decision to go home and die rather than comply with medical directives.

- An adult daughter's choices regarding caring for her invalid mother.

- A diabetic woman's choice of balancing care for herself and care for her family.

- A family's choice regarding withdrawing nutrition and life supports from a comatose relative.

In situations such as these, the NCMrs sought to help clients view the disease as an opportunity to know themselves better and to use the situation as a stimulus to realize a fuller sense of self.

Beginning and ending. The NCMrs are confronted with decisions regarding access to care that most nurses have not had to face: decisions regarding selection of clients *and* decisions to terminate service, at least for that phase of care. In traditional nursing services, the responsibility for initiating and terminating a nurse-client relationship usually has been defined by programmatic or reimbursement guidelines. For example, under Medicare guidelines, home health nursing services are terminated when the client no longer requires "skilled nursing" or no longer is homebound. In NCM at St. Mary's, these decisions regarding visit frequency are negotiated by the NCMr and client. In instances of intense ongoing need for nursing consultation, the NCMrs can easily fall into a codependent relationship with the client. One NCMr commented, "Hanging in there [for a long period of time] has paid off, but when doesn't it work? When can you let go?" Some of the signposts that the work is done are when the clients are able to cope with their situation, have resolved a particular decision (choice) or reached a plateaulike resting point, are able to handle community services on their own, or when death occurs.

RELATIONSHIP TO HOSPITAL STAFF

The need for communication between the NCMr and the hospital nursing staff is critical for integration and continuity of care. Initially, role relationships between the NCMrs and hospital nursing staff were sensitive, but with clarification of the expectations and complementarity of both roles, mutual respect was expressed for the contribution each makes to the client's welfare. Hospital nursing staff are becoming increasingly alert to cues that help from an NCMr is indicated, and the NCMrs are becoming increasingly aware of the importance of providing feedback regarding clients who have been referred to them by the hospital staff. The hospital nurses expressed the need to experience the benefit that accrued by referral of the client to the NCMr. When clients return to the hospital (and the cycle begins again), the NCMr shares relevant information with the hospital staff and participates in discharge planning.

Mutuality and exchange between the NCMrs and hospital nursing staff are enhanced by the NCMr's visibility on the hospital unit. NCMrs accomplished visibility in several ways: by spending regular time on the hospital units, by familiarizing staff with their total caseload by posting a list of their clients, by iden ifying the hospitalized clients being followed by an NCMr by placiu₅ the NCMr's name on the face sheet of the client's record, and by participating in discharge planning rounds.

LINKING THEORY AND PRACTICE

Newman: One of my initial objectives for visiting St. Mary's was to examine the relevance of my theory of health and nurse-client relationships to their practice. I quickly found that the intensity of the dialectic process required that I devote my full attention to allowing the nature of the NCMr's practice to emerge. Therefore, I set aside the objective of evaluating the relevance of my theory to practice until I had completed the interviews and the analysis of the data. This setting aside was not unlike bracketing, an element in phenomenological research. At the same time, the adoption of the hermeneutic dialectic stance permitted me the freedom to share my point of view as the construction of the practice emerged. The congruence of the emerging themes with my previous conceptualization of nursing practice was striking. The dimensions of the nurse-client relationships described by the NCMrs paralleled the characteristics of nursing and the nurse-client relationship described in my theory of health as expanding consciousness (Newman, 1986, 1989): (1) the nurse coming together with clients at critical choice points in their lives and participating with them in the process of expanding consciousness, (2) rhythmicity and timing in the relationship, (3) letting go of the need to direct the relationship, (4) pattern identification as an essential element in the process, and (5) personal transformation. There was no specific intent on the part of the NCMrs to "apply" my theory. Their practice was a *manifestation* of the theory.

Lamb and Michaels: In our work with Margaret, we became aware of the fit between our practice as NCMrs and her theory. Although we had an intuitive grasp of our work with clients, Margaret's theory provided a structure for explicating meaningful concepts and the process that evolves between nurse and client. The time spent exploring the interplay between the theory of expanding consciousness and our NCM practice provided us with a mirror for looking at our practice patterns and decisions. It uncovered a need to scrutinize our decisions and interactions with clients around pivotal issues, such as timing and frequency of visits. Although we had previously recognized the importance of timing, we realized that for NCM to achieve quality *and* cost-related goals, the timing and rhythm of interactions must be finely tuned. We began to talk about "stepping in and stepping back." We recognized that we must be attuned to cues that call for rapid intense intervention, as well as cues that reflect a plateau or resting period where the NCMr can reduce visit frequency and wait and watch for a while. We found that gauging the clients' health needs to the frequency and intensity of service requires timely assessment of dynamic patterns, and we recognized that our developing knowledge and skill could be guided by Margaret's theory.

Newman. Given the nature of cooperative inquiry, it is not surprising that the structure that emerged in this study reflected my interpretive framework. I am quite aware that it is not the only structure that could have emerged, but it is a valid one nevertheless. Another investigator might have viewed the NCMrs' practice in terms of caring or promoting self-care, and certainly those factors were present. I looked at it in terms of the mutual process of expanding consciousness through pattern recognition and facilitating choices, and those factors, too, were indeed present. The link between theory and practice was strengthened by the congruence of the language of the NCMrs with the language of the theory, as well as the mutual validation experienced by the NCMrs and me during the sharing of the data of their practice experiences in relation to the theory.

LINKING THE THEORY OF PRACTICE TO THE NURSING ENTERPRISE

The coming together of theory and practice is a first step in the definition and documentation of nursing practice needed to satisfy third-party payers. Nursing enterprise at St. Mary's is defined as the business of providing high-quality, cost-effective nursing services for a fee or by capitation. Moving into a capitated system for nurse case management (Schorr, 1990) has accelerated the need to incorporate theory into NCM. A commitment to quality outcomes combined with fiscal responsibility requires increasingly close attention to the process of care delivery. There is a need for efficient client pattern identification and matching of services to client's needs and choices. A recent contract has been enacted between a health maintenance organization (HMO) and NCM at St. Mary's, extending this quality of nursing service to an additional 400 clients. The theory-practice link facilitated contract negotiations by clarifying the distinctly complementary nature of the nursing service offered by NCM in relation to the medical services already offered by the HMO.

Central to the successful resolution of the reimbursement issue is recognition that nursing care emanates from a different paradigm than medical care. The usual acceptable measurable outcomes of the medical paradigm reflect a system based on cure rather than care. These outcomes often do not accurately reflect the effectiveness of nursing care. The criteria for reimbursement emanating from a nursing paradigm are based on the process of pattern recognition and successful resolution of clients' choices. To address this need for a different kind of documentation, the NCMrs at St. Mary's have begun to document their practice in terms of narrative summaries of the process that clients and nurses engage in during the resolution of long-term care situations. Studies are in progress to describe the process from the clients' point of view (Gerri Lamb & Joan Stempel, personal communication) and to compare the practice of the NCMrs with other models.

REFERENCES

Guba, E. G., & Lincoln, Y. S. (1989). *Fourth generation evaluation.* Newbury Park, CA: Sage.

Newman, M. A. (1986). *Health as expanding consciousness.* St. Louis: C. V. Mosby.

Newman, M. A. (1989). The spirit of nursing. *Holistic Nursing Practice, 3*(3), 1–6.

Schorr, T. M. (1990). Eyes on the future. Phyllis Ethridge, Nurse-run managed care? *American Journal of Nursing, 90*(10), 25.

CHAPTER TWENTY

The Professional Doctorate: Education for Professional Practice

Margaret A. Newman

IF ONE WERE to analyze public feeling about health and health care delivery, one might come to the conclusion that the public, in general, sees health care as the domain of the physician. The crisis in health delivery is attributed to the shortage of physicians. Federal health planning groups are composed primarily of physicians. And it is to the physician that the conscientious individual pays a yearly visit for a health examination.

At the same time, the public is becoming increasingly dissatisfied with the quality of the health care it is receiving. People seem to know there is something missing, but they are not quite sure what that is. At any rate, they are aware of the high cost of medical and hospital care and equally aware of the unavailability of physicians for everyday problems.

I believe that nursing has what the public is looking for. Because nursing is concerned with the everyday problems of living and has the knowledge and skill to fill the gap in the public's health needs, I believe that it can and should do so, in collaboration with other health

Reprinted with permission from article originally titled "The Professional Doctorate in Nursing: A Position Paper," *Nursing Outlook,* 23(11):704–706, 1975. Copyright: The American Journal of Nursing Co.

professionals. Nursing *has* what the public needs but it somehow has not succeeded in getting it to the public in sufficiently large and noticeable quantities.

Medical educators are becoming aware of the deficiencies in the traditional medical approach to health and are calling for changes in medical curricula to provide for ". . . doctors who are more humane, socially conscious, or liberally educated." They are recognizing the need to "teach the care of patients and not disease" (Heaney, 1974). These changes will certainly benefit the public; however, why should the public have to wait until these changes can be effected when there is a health professional already prepared in this way?

The focus of nursing education has, from the days of Florence Nightingale, been directed toward the individualized, personalized care of the patient, not the disease. Admittedly, nursing has at times strayed from its purpose, but great strides have been made in the last twenty years in identifying the knowledge needed for the health care of people at all stages of life and in preparing nursing practitioners who have this knowledge and can put it into action.

Why, then, has nursing not succeeded in demonstrating its value to the public? Nursing lacks both recognition for what it has to offer and authority for putting that knowledge into practice. If we are to fulfill our commitment to society and be true to ourselves in terms of actualizing our potential, we will have to claim the recognition and authority which are rightfully ours by virtue of our education and expertise. One way of getting recognition for the education many of our practitioners already have and of ensuring that future nursing practitioners have equal status with other major health professionals is to offer a professional doctorate—a Doctor of Nursing—as the degree obtained at the end of programs preparing professional practitioners.

This *professional* doctorate is not to be confused with an *academic* doctorate. The latter, the Ph.D., is an advanced research degree, preceded by basic (undergraduate) education in the field, and is intended to prepare scholars who will advance and teach the knowledge of the field. In contrast, a professional doctorate is a practice degree, similar to the Doctor of Medicine degree, and constitutes basic preparation for practice.

One of the arguments against this position is that nursing should not imitate medicine by offering a similar degree. However, medicine is not the only profession offering a professional doctorate. On the contrary, a number of the professions offer such a degree: law (J.D.), dentistry (D.D.S.), pharmacy (D.Ph.), and others. The content in programs leading to these degrees is comparable to what nursing students learn in a combination of the baccalaureate and master's programs and, in some instances, to what students are taught in baccalaureate programs alone. . . .

Another argument against the professional doctorate in nursing is that yet another degree in nursing would be further "muddying the water." This can be countered by pointing out that movement toward the professional doctorate will eliminate some of the confusion, rather than cause more, because there might then be less question among nurses as to who is prepared to be the professional practitioner.

The baccalaureate degree, supposedly our professional degree, is certainly no guarantee that one has really had a professional education in nursing. Some generic baccalaureate programs in nursing differ very little from technical programs. Other baccalaureate programs, based on the ladder concept, are being offered to RNs whose preparation was in technical programs, and the upper division courses in these programs are concerned more with leadership skills than with the science of nursing.

In addition, some nurses question how adequately even "good" baccalaureate programs prepare the professional practitioner, as evidenced by the droves of baccalaureate graduates returning to master's programs in order to obtain more clinical expertise or, as some have admitted, to escape the frustrating limitations placed on their activities in practice settings.

Perhaps we should consider that a four-year baccalaureate program is probably *not* sufficient to prepare the person for the level of independent practice needed and demanded by the public today. Then, rather than adding on another year or so to the baccalaureate program or even giving master's credit for some additional knowledge (which many educators have difficulty identifying other than as "broader and deeper"), we should perhaps plan a total and thoroughly integrated program. Such a program would clearly delineate the components needed for independent professional practice in nursing and grant a degree that is indicative of the student's preparation for practice and affords him status comparable to that enjoyed by other professional practitioners.

The current trend toward an interdisciplinary approach toward the teaching of health sciences provides further evidence of the similarities among curricula in all the health fields (Pellegrino, 1970). The proponents of this approach seek to identify the common educational needs of students in the major health professions, eliminate the duplication of courses from professional school to professional school, and offer the content which all students need in courses which they all take. In other words, there would no longer be a need for a physiology course for dental students and then another physiology course for nursing students and so on, if the content of the courses is the same.

In addition to providing a common science base, the interdisciplinary approach encourages each professional school to offer content from its own field that may be relevant to the needs of the others. The four major tracks of such a curriculum—dentistry, medicine, nursing, pharmacy—stem from a common base, with each profession having a focus appropriate to the service which it offers. Is it not reasonable that the degree awarded at the completion of each of these tracks should be comparable?

Lastly, the position of the Doctor of Nursing degree within the overall picture of nursing and nursing education must be considered. Obviously, in addition to the need for the independent nurse practitioner, there will continue to be a great need for nursing technicians and for supervisors and teachers of nursing technicians. The education of persons for all of these roles in nursing technology should be distinctly different from the education of persons for practice and teaching roles within nursing.

Part of the difficulty in differentiating between the two types of practice is that teachers in the two types of educational programs have similar educational backgrounds and are therefore not clear themselves about the difference between professional nursing and nursing technology. In some instances, the content of professional nursing practice is taught to people who want to become nursing technicians; in others, the reverse is true. Therefore, I would propose a separate educational track for persons whose career objectives relate to nursing technology rather than nursing. Each of these tracks contains continued opportunity for educational advancement, as shown in Table 20.1.

Even though a baccalaureate degree in nursing need not necessarily precede the D.N.* degree, perhaps—at least, in the transitional phase of such a program—a baccalaureate degree should be granted after completion of part of the program, and the D.N. after completion of the total program. This dual degree plan is offered in a number of other professional schools—for example, law and pharmacy.

Adoption of the above plan would re-emphasize the need to distinguish the two types of practitioner and to sanction both levels of practice with a licensing law for each level. Since the professional practitioner will be functioning directly with people in the context of their families, regardless of the setting or the focus of the activity, an appropriate name for this practitioner might be "Family Nurse." Perhaps this title would communicate to the public that there is someone to fill the gap in their health needs that has been made apparent by the absence of family physicians. In the case of

---

* The Doctor of Nursing degree is now more usually referred to as the N.D. degree.

Table 20.1   Proposed Educational Tracks

Nursing		Nursing Technology	
Objective	*Degree*	*Objective*	*Degree*
Practice	Doctor of Nursing	Practice	Associate of Arts
Teaching and/ or research	Ph.D.	Supervision	Baccalaureate degree (based on ladder concept, complementing A.A. with courses relating to leadership ability and broader view of health)
		Teaching	Master's degree* in teaching of nursing technology

* Currently an academic doctorate is the usual requirement.

this new nurse practitioner, there would again be a family "doctor," but this time the doctor would be a nurse.

I do not mean to imply in any way, however, that the family nurse would be taking on the role of the physician. On the contrary, the family nurse would be fulfilling nursing's commitment to family health with a title that would reflect the nurse's abilities and responsibilities.

In summary, I believe that nursing now has the knowledge and skill to provide the type of health care needed by society. I believe that part of the reason that this product has not been delivered is lack of recognition, both within and outside nursing's ranks, of nursing's ability to deliver it. I believe that adoption of a professional degree similar to that awarded in the other major health professions will be a step toward assuring an appropriate educational base for the practitioner and claiming for nursing the recognition and status needed for the task.

REFERENCES

Heaney, R. P. (1974). Interdisciplinary integration in health sciences curricula. *Trans. New York Academy of Science, 36,* 324–332.

Pellegrino, E. D. (1970). Medical practice and the new curricula. *Journal of the American Medical Association, 213,* 748–752.

Retrospective:
Theory for Nursing Practice

Margaret A. Newman

In May 1992 I celebrated with my undergraduate class of 1962 the thirty years we have been engaged in nursing. It prompted me to think about what has changed in nursing during that time . . . what has stayed the same. I have devoted most of my professional life to trying to find answers to questions I was faced with as an undergraduate student, questions regarding what knowledge guided nursing: the theory of nursing practice. I will reminisce a bit about nursing's development as a discipline over the past 30 years.

In the fall of 1961 I happened to read an article that set the direction for my professional work. The article was "The Significance of Nursing Care" by Dorothy Johnson. She said basically that nursing was different from medicine; therefore the underlying knowledge was different. That seems simple now but was revolutionary then. She saw the goal of nursing practice as helping people find a sense of equilibrium in the experience of illness, and in her article, she began to explicate her theory of dynamic equilibrium.

Reprinted with permission from Nursing Science Quarterly, 7(4):153–157, 1994. Based on paper presented at Symposium 3—Developing Knowledge for Nursing Practice, University of Rhode Island, October, 1992.

D. Johnson's (1961) article was like a bolt of light piercing the darkness and confusion that I had been experiencing as a student in trying to apply what I was learning to nursing practice. What I was learning in school was mostly medical knowledge: the description and treatment of disease, with a little nursing care thrown in, mostly as a tag-on. But prior to entering nursing, I had experienced what it was like to be the primary caregiver for my mother, who was experiencing a long-term debilitating disease, and what Johnson was saying about nursing made sense to me. It fit what I had tried to accomplish in my mother's care. Based on this experience, I sensed on some subliminal level the essence of nursing. As a nursing student, I had fleeting glimpses of the significance of nursing care as I learned alongside a very intelligent, intuitive, compassionate nursing instructor. But the nature of that nursing knowledge was elusive, and I did not know where to turn on my own to concentrate on the study of nursing. I could not articulate nursing as a discipline. I recognized the necessity of having a discipline as part of nursing's status as a profession, but I did not know how to describe the body of knowledge that characterized nursing as a discipline. D. Johnson's (1961) article on the significance of nursing care opened the door for the odyssey that has occupied my professional life.

CHARTING THE COURSE FOR THE DISCIPLINE

The question that challenged me over 30 years ago—what is the theory of nursing practice?—is still relevant. We have come a long way since then. I will try to pinpoint some of the steps along the way, and some earlier ones.

From 1952 through the mid-'70s a number of conceptual models based on theories from other disciplines applicable to nursing practice were set forth: for example, theories of interpersonal relations (Peplau,

1952), communication (Orlando, 1961), biological and social adaptation (Roy, 1976). These models represented a definite shift from emphasis on medical science to emphasis on the interpersonal process involved in nursing and recognition of the active participation of the client in the health-illness process.

The research of that early period, however, was based primarily on a problem-oriented approach drawn from practice. We knew we needed to do research, but we did not know much about how theory related to research. We could see problems in practice that needed to be studied, and so we identified a problem, searched for an explanation (theory), and then tested a solution to the problem. In that period we were emulating the research paradigm of the biophysical sciences, in which the experimental method was dominant. It was recognized that not all of the problems of clinical nursing could be solved by an experimental approach; therefore, exploratory, experiential studies were undertaken but were considered valid only as stepping stones to more controlled research.

Martha Rogers' work, which became prominent in the late sixties and early seventies, represented a turning point in identifying the substance of nursing theory. Rogers (1970) rejected a practice-oriented approach to the development of nursing knowledge. She insisted that we *start* from theory, from a set of basic assumptions about the phenomenon she identified as the center of nursing practice: the phenomenon of the human being. She introduced a revolutionary, unitary way of viewing the human being by stipulating assumptions such as wholeness, pattern, and unidirectionality: the assumption of wholeness meaning that nursing's focus is the person as a whole and that nursing science must address knowledge of the whole; the assumption of pattern being that pattern identifies the person and depicts the innovative wholeness of the person's mutual, unidirectional evolution within an open environmental field (Rogers, 1970).

The purpose of Rogers' framework was to outline a distinctly different science—*nursing* science—based on a holistic view of the human being as one with the environment. She, too, clearly asserted that the knowledge of nursing differed from that of other disciplines and that we could not expect to develop this knowledge by pursuing the concepts and methods of other disciplines.

This call for a distinctly different discipline was an important insight on the part of early theorists. It was easy to accept their insistence on a new science, but it was not easy to envision it. We had not seen it before. We were immersed in the knowledge of a particulate world seen through the eyes of other disciplines and could not imagine anything beyond that. The prevailing scientific paradigm was one that assumed that it was valid to analyze organisms (including human beings) into parts, reduce those elements to neatly measurable entities, control and manipulate the parts, and then try to extrapolate to the whole based on knowledge of the parts. For most of us, that was the standard against which all research was judged. It seemed crazy and unreal to accept a paradigm that stipulated the necessity of looking at the whole. Walker (1971) suggested that Rogers was asking for more than science could give, that is, that Rogers was asking for the experience of the phenomenon rather than the description. I'm sure not even Walker knew then how relevant a forecast she had made of the nursing science that was to evolve. In defense of Rogers' call for holism, I suggested then that we could carefully select holistic parameters that could be described and measured and fit into the methods of normal science (Newman, 1979), but my attempts to do this yielded results that did not satisfy the need for a holistic science. Both Walker and I were trying to deal with the concept of holism within the context of a particulate science. The square pegs/round holes phenomenon.

ONTOLOGY VIS-À-VIS EPISTEMOLOGY

In spite of the call to holism, and the acceptance of holism as a philosophical foundation of the nursing profession, the bulk of the research in nursing, both then and now, has been structured within a scientific paradigm based on causal analysis and predictability (Newman, 1992; Reynolds, 1988). The prevailing scientific paradigm in nursing today attempts to combine the holistic values of the profession with the objectivity and predictability of a post-positivist philosophy. Sime, Corcoran-Perry, and I have labeled it an interactive-integrative paradigm, a term that depicts the interactive nature of the multiple phenomena involved in the study of the human experience and designates integration as the way in which change takes place—a convergence of parts to make up the whole (Newman, Sime, & Corcoran-Perry, 1991). This paradigm holds to the positivist beliefs of objectivity, control, and predictability but acknowledges the subjectivity, multidimensionality, and context-dependent nature of the human experience. The centrality of objectivity and predictability to this paradigm are the key points that differentiate it from one that is truly holistic. If these beliefs are taken as truth, as reality, then a paradigm that embraces inability to control and non-predictability is clearly non-truth, non-reality.

Yet an increasing number of nursing scientists have realized that the phenomenon of nursing practice is not characterized by prediction and control. Gradually we have begun to see that knowledge based on methods that separate and isolate entities does not reflect nursing phenomena. Bohm (1980) pointed out the fallacy of fragmented thinking: "Some might say 'Wholeness is only an ideal, toward which we should perhaps strive.' . . . what should be said is that wholeness is what is real, and that fragmentation is the response of this whole" (p. 7) to fragmentary thinking. What is needed is not an integration or an imposed unity of parts, but an implicit grasp of the whole.

STATUS OF THE DISCIPLINE

Meanwhile, during the '70s and '80s, we were preoccupied with our status as a discipline and turned to learning *about* theory per se as a means to the development of the discipline. We were involved in discussions of the nature of theory and what makes it nursing theory. We made significant strides in establishing our credibility as a discipline, as evidenced by the expansion of doctoral programs in nursing and the increasing federal support for research.

But the question of what is the focus of the discipline of nursing has not been resolved. The wide range of foci of the work conducted by nurse theorists and researchers is apparent. But, simply having a nurse as the author is not enough to assure that the work contributes to the discipline. We must question how these different emphases relate to the discipline of nursing and, more specifically, whether or not the research findings make a difference in practice.

To this end, several of us at the University of Minnesota, recognizing that the emphasis of our research was widely different, decided to try to determine what these varied approaches to nursing research had in common (Newman, Sime, & Corcoran-Perry, 1991). At one point, I concluded that the differences among us were a matter of paradigm, the scientific paradigm that guides one's investigations. People working out of different paradigms see things differently and arrive at different conclusions, sometimes even with the same data.

The question of paradigm certainly is a factor. But as we pursued this overall issue, we were confronted with more basic questions: What is the focus of our discipline? What do we need to know in order to practice nursing? The paradigm issue became peripheral, at least for the moment, to the question of focus. The discipline of nursing is the study of what?

Over a century ago, Florence Nightingale (1992) had said that "the laws of nursing were the same as the laws of health," (p. 6, facsimile of original work) both of which were unknown. She meant health as the whole, of which disease and illness are parts. In the '70s and '80s a large number of theorists and researchers picked up Nightingale's torch and began to pursue knowledge of *health* as central to nursing (Newman, 1992; Pender, 1984). At the same time, an equally compelling cadre of theorists focused on *caring* as the essence of nursing (Benner, 1988; Leininger, 1990; Morse, Solberg, Neander, Bottorff, & Johnson, 1990; Watson, 1988). These two areas of theory and research—health and caring—emerged in the '80s as major emphases of the professional discipline that is nursing. But neither alone is sufficient to specify the focus of the discipline. Neither is the exclusive domain of nursing. But the two taken together, caring in the human health experience, specify a phenomenon of inquiry and a domain of service that nursing may call its own.

Specifying the health component as the human health experience clearly distinguishes the focus from that of medicine and encompasses the vast array of health experiences not specifically associated with disease. Specifying caring as an essential component of the discipline makes clear the profession's commitment to the well-being of society. This integrated emphasis takes into account circumscription of the aspect of the knowledge domain of human experience for which nursing is responsible (the human health experience), and the nature of the relationship that nursing assumes in terms of its commitment to society (caring). Together these dimensions define the focus of the discipline.

If we can accept this focus, we know what we need to know. Theories of nursing, the science of nursing, must address the complex, holistic dynamic of caring in the human health experience. This focus requires a scientific paradigm that embraces a unitary, transformative perspective.

When Sime, Corcoran-Perry, and I began work on the question of how our disparate research relates to nursing, we thought of ourselves as each representing different paradigms, but as we came to accept the disciplinary focus of nursing as caring in the human health experience, each of us became convinced of the need for a paradigm that would take us beyond the analysis of related constructs and embrace the unitary, self-organizing nature of the human being. Even the most "scientific" among us shared examples of her practice and research that could not be controlled and predicted—phenomena that demanded this unitary, transformative view. An important assumption of this view, supported by Prigogine's (Prigogine, Allen, & Herman, 1977) theory of dissipative structures, is that at various points in the process, change is unpredictable. The living system is part of a giant fluctuation of on-going transformations, and the direction it ultimately chooses to pursue cannot be predicted. Knowledge based on the prevailing paradigm of objectivity and control is relevant to one phase of this process but not sufficient for a full elaboration and understanding of the nursing phenomenon.

We have come to see nursing as a process of relationship that co-evolves as a function of the interpenetration of the evolving fields of the nurse, client, and environment in a self-organizing, unpredictable way. We recognize the need for "process wisdom" (Vaill, 1984–1985), the ability to come from the center of our truth and act in the immediate moment. Not only is our science a *human* science, but within the context of a practice discipline, it is a science of *praxis*. This kind of theory is *embodied* in the investigator-nurse. It informs the situation being addressed by making a difference in the situation, as well as being informed by the data of the situation.

The focus issue and the paradigm issue are interconnected. The paradigm issue is one that has been hard to recognize because whatever paradigm guides one's thinking *is reality* for that person. The nature of a paradigm is so pervasive and deeply embedded that it becomes normative. It determines what is important. It is like a culture—shared knowledge—and adherents cannot imagine any other way to behave.

SHIFTING TO A NEW PARADIGM

How does one then shift to a new paradigm? A paradigm shift is an equally difficult phenomenon to grasp. My experience went like this: I was aware for a long time of a vague feeling of discontent, a feeling that things didn't quite fit, and yet I was determined to make them fit.

I ignored the fact that I was deceiving myself: I was supporting a unitary theoretical framework on the one hand but conducting research based on assumptions contradictory to the theory. Finally I began to allow the assumptions of the theory to determine the methods of the research. I let go of the need to control and manipulate and shifted into a mode of being fully present, authentically myself—seeking to know and trusting that the knowledge inherent in the situation would emerge. One day I felt the relief and joy of method congruent with theory.

My approach to the development of theory for practice has followed the pattern outlined above. It started with problem identification—a clinical problem identification—followed by a search for some theoretical rationale to support a hypothesis, which then identified an action aimed at a desired health outcome. As I became clearer in terms of my own philosophical-theoretical stance, I began to construct a theoretical set of propositions from which to derive hypotheses. Both of these approaches yielded information that was relevant to nursing practice but was not comprehensive enough to *structure* the practice. That is, the findings could be applied in practice but were not comprehensive enough to guide the whole of practice.

The current phase of my work began with the study of pattern. There was a need to be able to identify the pattern of a person. Pattern was a basic assumption of my theoretical position. Pattern of the whole was the unit of knowledge called for by the initial work of the nurse theorists' designation of a framework for nursing diagnosis (Roy, 1982). I had learned through trial and error that trying to identify pattern by adding up or even synthesizing bits of information was not workable. One had to somehow glimpse the whole, a phenomenon that sometimes occurs in practitioners' intuitive leaps. I quit asking for bits and pieces of information from clients and began asking clients to tell their stories, to describe what was important to them, what was most meaningful in their lives (Newman, 1987). In the data that resulted, I was able to glimpse the pattern of the whole from the stories of their lives. The pattern of the unfolding relationships of their lives was interpreted in terms of the theory of health as expanding consciousness (Newman, 1986; Newman & Moch, 1991). This work focuses on the wholeness of the person's experience. There is no attempt to control the response. The data speaks for itself when viewed in terms of the theory. The support for the theory is not exclusive. What one sees in the data depends on the theoretical perspective from which one views the data; therefore, the same data could be used to support other theories.

To examine the relevancy of this theory in practice, I engaged in a dialogue with a group of nurses whose practice appeared to be philosophically congruent with my own position. A description of their practice experience supported key elements of my theory: the importance of pattern recognition, timing, and mutuality of the nurse-client relationship. The theory was not something external to the nurse that was applied; *the theory was lived by the nurse* and manifested in the nurse's practice. The more expanded the consciousness of the nurses, the more readily they were able to enter into a transformative relationship with clients (Newman, Lamb, & Michaels, 1991).

Sometime during the past 30 years, then, a paradigm shift has occurred in nursing. There is evidence in the nursing literature of a shift from a medical model to a holistic model (M. B. Johnson, 1990). There is evidence of the commonly shared themes of several contemporary nursing theories: themes of holism, process, and self-transcendence (Sarter, 1988). The science of nursing is no longer pre-paradigmatic. We have crossed the threshold of becoming a science. Our paradigm embraces the whole of the human experience in an evolving, self-organizing world. This calls for methods that will allow us to be participant-observers in the phenomenon of nursing: caring in the human health experience. Knowledge emanating from the study of this focus empowers nurses in practice. Theory for nursing practice is more than the application of single-dimension theories in specific practice situations. It is a matter of *the nurse's being transformed by the theory and thereby becoming a transforming partner in interaction with clients.*

When asked in 1978 what I thought nursing was, I said that the goal of nursing is not necessarily to make people well, or to prevent their becoming ill, but to assist people to utilize the power that is within as they evolve toward higher levels of consciousness. It has taken almost 30 years to figure out how to do that . . . and I am still learning.

REFERENCES

Benner, P. (1988, October). *Nursing as a caring profession.* Paper presented at meeting of the American Academy of Nursing, Kansas City, MO.

Bohm, D. (1980). *Wholeness and the implicate order.* London: Routledge & Kegan Paul.

Johnson, D. (1961). The significance of nursing care. *American Journal of Nursing, 61*(11), 63–66.

Johnson, M. B. (1990). The holistic paradigm in nursing: The diffusion of an innovation. *Research in Nursing and Health, vol. 13,* 129–139.

Leininger, M. (1990). Historic and epistemologic dimensions of care and caring with future directions. In J. Stevenson and T. Tripp-Reimer (Eds.), *Proceedings of a Wingspread Conference: Knowledge about care and caring.* Kansas City, MO: American Academy of Nursing.

Morse, J. M., Solberg, S. M., Neander, W. L., Bottorff, J. L., & Johnson, J. L. (1990). Concepts of caring and caring as a concept. *Advances in Nursing Science, 13*(1), 1–14.

Newman, M. A. (1979). *Theory development in nursing.* Philadelphia: Davis.

Newman, M. A. (1986). *Health as expanding consciousness.* St. Louis: Mosby.

Newman, M. A. (1987). Patterning. In M. Duffy & N. J. Pender (Eds.), *Proceedings of a Wingspread Conference: Conceptual issues in health promotion* (pp. 36–50). Indianapolis: Sigma Theta Tau.

Newman, M. A. (1992). Health conceptualizations. *Annual Review of Nursing Research, 9,* 221–243.

Newman, M. A., Lamb, G. S., & Michaels, C. (1991). Nurse case management: The coming together of theory and practice. *Nursing & Health Care, 12*(8), 404–408.

Newman, M. A., & Moch, S. D. (1991). Life patterns of persons with coronary heart disease. *Nursing Science Quarterly, 4,* 161–167.

Newman, M. A., Sime, A. M., & Corcoran-Perry, S. A. (1991). The focus of the discipline. *Advances in Nursing Science, 14*(1), 1–6.

Nightingale, F. (1992). *Notes on nursing: What it is and what it is not.* Commemorative Edition. Philadelphia: Lippincott.

Orlando, I. (1961). *The dynamic nurse-patient relationship.* New York: Putnam.

Pender, N. J. (1984). Health promotion and illness prevention. *Annual Review of Nursing Research, 3,* 83–106.

Peplau, H. E. (1952). *Interpersonal relations in nursing.* New York: Putnam.

Prigogine, I., Allen, P. M., & Herman, R. (1977). Long-term trends and the evolution of complexity. In E. Laszlo & J. Bierman (Eds.), *Goals in a global community: The original background papers for goals for mankind: Vol. I. Studies on the conceptual foundation* (pp. 1–63). New York: Pergamon.

Reynolds, C. L. (1988). The measurement of health in nursing research. *Advances in Nursing Science, 10*(4), 23–31.

Rogers, M. E. (1970). *An introduction to the theoretical basis of nursing.* Philadelphia: Davis.

Roy, C. (1976). *Introduction to nursing: An adaptation model.* Englewood Cliffs, NJ: Prentice-Hall.

Roy, C. (1982). Theoretical framework for classification of nursing diagnosis (1978). In M. J. Kim & D. A. Moritz (Eds.), *Classification of nursing diagnoses:* Proceedings of the 3rd and 4th National Conferences (pp. 215–221). New York: McGraw Hill.

Sarter, B. (1988). Philosophical sources of nursing theory. *Nursing Science Quarterly, 1,* 52–59.

Vaill, P. B. (1984–1985). Process wisdom for a new age. *Re-Vision, 7*(2), 39–49.

Walker, L. O. (1971). Toward a clearer understanding of the concept of nursing theory. *Nursing Research, 20*(5), 428–435.

Watson, M. J. (1988). New dimensions of human caring theory. *Nursing Science Quarterly, 1,* 175–181.

Prospective:
Into the 21st Century

Margaret Newman

Written on the occasion to the 25th anniversary celebration at the School of Nursing. The Pennsylvania State University. (April 1993) Adapted for this volume.

> The 21st century is upon us.
> We are at a breakpoint
> In the development of
> Nursing's contribution
> To the health of society.
>
> We are at the breakpoint
> Of entering an integrating cycle
> Of development
> As a professional discipline.
> We know who we are
> As a profession
> As a discipline
> And the world is beginning to know
> It needs us.
>
> Around 1980
> There was a book,
> *We Are the Earthquake Generation,*
> About predictions
> Of seismologists and psychics
> Scientists and seers
> Who said that as we approach the 21st century

Excerpted and reprinted with permission from *Nursing Science Quarterly*, 7(1):44–46. 1994.

We will experience increasing
Physical disturbances:
Earthquakes and volcanic eruptions,
Hurricanes and floods,
And not only that,
Social and political disturbances
Changing the way the people of the world
Relate to each other.

We *are* the earthquake generation.
Things are breaking up
And washing away
All around us.
Violent storms
Just this past year
Are very much with us.
In the last decade
Changes have taken place
That have transformed the world.

The Berlin Wall has come down;
The Soviet Union has been dissolved;
Eastern Europe has thrown off the mantle
Of Soviet Communist dictatorship
And now people in all those places
Are experiencing the disorganization
Of the evolving process.

With instant worldwide communication
We are closer to and aware of
The anguish
And violence
Of long-suppressed hatred.
We are aware of the deprivation
Of starving people
In Africa
And Bosnia
And other parts of the world
Including, but sometimes not as evident,
Those in our own backyards.

We are faced with an increasing awareness
Of the abuse in our society:
Abuse of children
Abuse by children
Abuse of the elderly
Abuse of women
Abuse of people in the workplace
Abuse of nurses.

This is not a pretty picture
But we can look forward
To the changes taking place.
As the walls of the old structures
Are crumbling,
There is hope for a new structure
Of government, business, education.
There is hope for a new structure
Of health care.

Chaos theory
Depicts a system that fluctuates
In a so-called "normal" repetitive pattern
For a while
Until some precipitating factor
Disturbs the system and
Catapults it into disorganization
From which
A new, higher form of organization
Emerges.

The author of *Earthquake Generation*
Predicted that by the year 2000
We would be moving into a system
That would value the development
Of Individuals
More than the maintenance
Of governmental structure.
Our present government
Is beginning to recognize
The importance

Of everyone
Having access to health care.
In these times I am pleased to be a nurse,
Pleased because Nursing
Will play a major role
In the health care system
That will emerge
From the current rubble.

I pray that we will be ready
To step to the forefront
As the health needs of people
Are put first
Above the greed, status-seeking, and hierarchy
Of our present system.

What are the people's needs?

Talk to an old woman who has had cancer,
Among many other physical maladies,
And she will tell you of the
Lack of connectedness of her life,
Of the inability to experience her own
Warmth and caring.

Talk to a young middle-aged man
With coronary heart disease
And he will tell you
About the missed opportunities in his life
About feeling always in the bind
Of pleasing others
And finding it difficult
To express himself.

Talk to a young man with AIDS
And he will tell you
About his loss of friends and family.
He will tell you that
He regards the virus
As a friend
That is helping him
To know himself and others.

Many who come to the attention
Of the current medical system
Will tell you of
Their deprived childhoods,
Childhoods during which they were
Alienated by alcoholic parents
Separated from their peers by chronic disease
Physically and psychologically abused.

So, you say, let's turn our attention
To the children of this world
So that they can be nurtured
Early in life,
And you ask the young, single mother
Who has no job
And no skills for getting a job,
What is important to her.
She will tell you
"I need to be me."
She is saying that
She needs the opportunity to become
The person
She can be
For herself and her own needs
And for the nurturing
Of her children.

Václav Havel has said that
Everyone needs a private place
To find one's authenticity.

Nursing has a responsibility
To find ways to
Nurture
The children
And their parents
And their parents' parents.

Nursing can do this.
We have accepted the commitment of a profession
That regards caring as a moral imperative.

We have a long tradition of caring,
Our discipline focuses on the knowledge of caring
In the human health experience,
A phenomenon
That goes beyond curing of disease.

What we need is the commitment to act.

It is time for
A parting with the past.
It is time to
Replace the anchor of the past
With the pull of the future.

We are in the process of creating
A shared vision.
In order to do so
It is necessary
To connect all parts of the system,
To integrate the similar
And the dissimilar
Unleashing the power of creativity.

The future vision
Draws from the past
But is not held back by it.

How do we do this?

Jose Arguelles says:
Stand in the center of your truth.

George Land says:
Organizations and nations
Don't change
Only individuals change
And that involves
Knowing who you are:
"When you know what you care about,
What you love,
What you have passion about,

You have discovered the deep truth
About who you are
And can fashion these gifts
Into something original."

The power of future pull
Is in knowing your purpose
And vision
And in bringing about
Circumstances in which
Everyone can win!

An important element
In the integrative cycle is
Eliminating judgments,
Which allows us to let go
Of the barriers that separate us
From people and events
That could bring new potentials
Into our lives.

By eliminating judgments
We can shift to
Connectedness
And the capacity to love.

We are committed to healing others.
Can we be committed to healing ourselves?
Our relationships?
Our society?
This requires an opening of our hearts
To ourselves and to one another.

The place to begin
Is at home.
David Bohm said we should
Form dialogue groups
Of people
From different perspectives,
A microcosm of the world.

And that we talk together
DIALOGUE
Meaning flowing through.
And through the process
Our many thoughts
Become one thought
A coherent thought
That has the power and clarity
Of a laser beam.

The power of our beam
Will coalesce with the power
Of other beams
Round the world
To enlighten the world.

We are indeed the earthquake generation.

Some of the ideas expressed were drawn from the following publications:

Bohm, D. (1992). On dialogue. *Noetic Sciences Review, 23,* 16–18.

Land, G., & Jarman, B. (1992). *Breakpoint and beyond.* New York: Harper Business.

Goodman, J. (1979). *We are the earthquake generation.* New York: Berkley.

Appendix

Author Publications
1966–1994

JOURNALS

Newman, M. A. (1994). Theory for nursing practice. *Nursing Science Quarterly, 7*(4), 153–157.

Newman, M. A. (1994). Into the 21st century. *Nursing Science Quarterly, 7*(1), 44–46.

Lamendola, F. P., & Newman, M. A. (1994). The paradox of HIV/AIDS as expanding consciousness. *Advances in Nursing Science, 16*(3), 13–21.

Newman, M. A. (1992). Prevailing paradigms in nursing. *Nursing Outlook, 40*(1), 10–13, 32.

Newman, M. A. (1991). Health conceptualizations. *Annual Review of Nursing Research,* Vol. 9, 221–243.

Newman, M. A., & Moch, S. D. (1991). Life patterns of persons with coronary heart disease. *Nursing Science Quarterly, 4*(4), 161–167.

Newman, M. A., Sime, A. M., & Corcoran-Perry, S. A. (1991). The focus of the discipline of nursing. *Advances in Nursing Science, 14*(1), 1–6.

Newman, M. A., Lamb, G. S., & Michaels, C. (1991). Nurse case management: The coming together of theory and practice. *Nursing & Health Care, 12*(8), 404–408.

Newman, M. A. (1991). Commentary: Research as practice. *Nursing Science Quarterly, 4*(3), 100–101.

Newman, M. A. (1990). Toward an integrative model of professional practice. *Journal of Professional Nursing, 6,* 167–173.

Newman, M. A. (1990). Newman's theory of health as praxis. *Nursing Science Quarterly, 3*(1), 37–41.

Newman, M. A. (1989). The spirit of nursing. *Holistic Nursing Practice, 3*(3), 1–6.

Newman, M. A. (1987). Aging as increasing complexity. *Journal of Gerontological Nursing, 13*(9), 16–18.

Butrin, J. A., & Newman, M. A. (1986). Health promotion in Zaire: Time perspective and cerebral hemispheric dominance as relevant factors. *Public Health Nursing, 3,* 183–191.

Newman, M. A., & Autio, S. (1986). Nursing in the world of DRGs and prospective payment. *CURA Reporter, 16*(5), 1–7.

Portonova, M., Young, E., & Newman, M. A. (1984). Elderly women's attitudes toward sexual activity among their peers. *Health Care for Women International, 5,* 289–298.

Newman, M. A. (1984). Nursing diagnosis: Looking at the whole. *American Journal of Nursing, 84,* 1496–1499.

Newman, M. A., & Gaudiano, J. K. (1984). Depression as an explanation for decreased subjective time in the elderly. *Nursing Research, 33,* 137–139.

Newman, M. A. (1983). Editorial. *Advances in Nursing Science, 5*(2), x–xi.

Newman, M. A. (1982). What differentiates clinical research? *Image, 14,* 86–88.

Newman, M. A. (1982). Time as an index of consciousness with age. *Nursing Research, 31,* 290–293.

Newman, M. A. & O'Brien, R. A. (1978). Experiencing the research process via computer simulation. *Image, 10,* 5–9.

Newman, M. A. (1976). Movement tempo and the experience of time. *Nursing Research, 25,* 273–279.

Newman, M. A. (1975). The professional doctorate in nursing: A position paper. *Nursing Outlook, 23,* 704–706.

Newman, M. A. (1972). Nursing's theoretical evolution. *Nursing Outlook, 20,* 449–453.

Newman, M. A. (1972). Time estimation in relation to gait tempo. *Perceptual and Motor Skills, 34,* 359–366.

Newman, M. A. (1966). Identifying patient needs in short-span nurse-patient relationships. *Nursing Forum, 5*(1), 76–86.

REVIEWS

Newman, M. A. (1991). [Review of Lowenberg, J. S., *Caring and responsibility: The crossroads between holistic practice and traditional medicine*]. *Journal of Professional Nursing, 7*(5), 319–320.

Newman, M. A. (1991). [Review of Barrett, E. A. M. (Ed.), *Visions of Rogers' science-based nursing*]. *Nursing Science Quarterly, 4*(1), 41–42.

Newman, M. A. (1987). Commentary [Y. Nojima et al., Perception of time among Japanese inpatients]. *Western Journal of Nursing Research, 9,* 299–300.

Newman, M. A. (1984). [Review of *Annual review of nursing research,* Vol. I, 1983]. *American Journal of Nursing,* 84, 1437–1438.

BOOKS, MONOGRAPHS AND CHAPTERS IN BOOKS

Newman, M. A. (1994). *Health as expanding consciousness.* 2nd Ed. New York: National League for Nursing.

Newman, M. A. (1992). Nightingale's vision of nursing theory and health. In F. Nightingale, *Notes on nursing.* Commemorative Edition. Philadelphia: Lippincott.

Newman, M. A. (1992). Nursing's theoretical evolution. In L. H. Nicoll (Ed.), *Perspectives in nursing theory* (pp. 77–84). Philadelphia: Lippincott.

Newman, M. A. (1990). Shifting to higher consciousness. In M. Parker (Ed.), *Nursing theories in practice* (pp. 129–139). New York: National League for Nursing.

Newman, M. A. (1990). Nursing paradigms and realities. In N. L. Chaska (Ed.), *The nursing profession: turning points* (pp. 230–235). St. Louis: Mosby.

Newman, M. A. (1990). Professionalism: myth or reality. In N. L. Chaska (Ed.), *The nursing profession: turning points* (pp. 49–52). St. Louis: Mosby.

Newman, M. A. (1987). Nursing's emerging paradigm: The diagnosis of pattern. In A. M. McLane (Ed.) *Classification of Nursing Diagnoses,* Proceedings of the Seventh Conference, North American Nursing Diagnosis Association (pp. 53–60). St. Louis: C. V. Mosby.

Newman, M. A. (1987). Patterning. In M. Duffy and N. J. Pender (Eds.), *Conceptual issues in health promotion, Report of Proceedings of a Wingspread Conference* (pp. 36–50). Indianapolis: Sigma Theta Tau.

Newman, M. A., & Autio, S. (1986). *Nursing in a prospective payment system health care environment.* Minneapolis: University of Minnesota School of Nursing.

Newman, M. A. (1986). *Health as expanding consciousness.* St. Louis: C. V. Mosby.

Newman, M. A. (1986). Nursing's theoretical evolution. In L. H. Nicoll (Ed.), *Perspectives on nursing theory* (pp. 72–78). Boston: Little, Brown & Co.

Newman, M. A. (1983). Newman's health theory. In I. Clements & F. Roberts (Eds.), *Family health: A theoretical approach to nursing care* (pp. 161–175). New York: John Wiley.

Newman, M. A. (1983). Nursing's theoretical evolution. In T. A. Duespohl (Ed.), *Nursing in transition* (pp. 15–24). Rockville, MD: Aspen.

Newman, M. A. (1983). The continuing revolution: A history of nursing science. In N. L. Chaska (Ed.), *The nursing profession: A time to speak* (pp. 385–393). New York: McGraw-Hill.

Roy, C., Rogers, M. E., Fitzpatrick, J. J., Newman, M. A., & Orem, D. E. (1982). Nursing diagnosis and nursing theory. In M. J. Kim & D. A. Moritz (Eds.), *Classification of nursing diagnosis* (pp. 215–231). New York: McGraw-Hill.

Feild, L., & Newman, M. A. (1982). Clinical application of the unitary man framework: Case study analysis. In M. J. Kim & D. A. Moritz (Eds.), *Classification of nursing diagnosis* (pp. 249–263). New York: McGraw-Hill.

Newman, M. A. (1981). The meaning of health. In G. E. Laskar (Ed.), *Applied systems research and cybernetics: Vol. 4. Systems research in health care, biocybernetics and ecology* (pp. 1739–1743). New York: Pergamon.

Newman, M. A. (1979). *Theory development in nursing.* Philadelphia: F. A. Davis. (Japanese rights assigned to Gendasha Publishing Company, Tokyo, 1986.)

Downs, F. S., & Newman, M. A. (Eds.). (1977). *A source book for nursing research* (2nd ed.). Philadelphia: F. A. Davis.

Downs, F. S., & Newman, M. A. (1977). Elements of a research critique. In F. S. Downs & M. A. Newman (Eds.), *A source book of nursing research* (2nd ed., pp. 1–12). Philadelphia: F. A. Davis.

Downs, F. S., & Newman, M. A. (Eds.). (1973). *A source book of nursing research.* Philadelphia: F. A. Davis.

Newman, M. A. (1973). Identifying patient needs in short-span nurse-patient relationships. In M. E. Auld & L. H. Birum (Eds.), *The challenge of nursing* (pp. 98–103). St. Louis: Mosby.

Index

Other Books of Interest from NLN Press

Book Title	Pub. No.	Price	NLN Member Price
☐ **Health As Expanding Consciousness (2nd ed.)** *By Margaret A. Newman*	14-2626	$35.95	$31.95
☐ **Illuminations: The Human Becoming Theory in Practice and Research** *Edited by Rosemarie Rizzo Parse*	15-2670	35.95	31.95
☐ **Rogers' Scientific Art of Nursing Practice** *Edited by Mary Madrid &* *Elizabeth Manhart Barrett*	15-2610	39.95	35.95
☐ **Visions of Rogers' Science-Based Nursing** *Edited by Elizabeth Manhart Barrett*	15-2285	40.95	36.95
☐ **Patterns of Nursing Theories in Practice** *Edited by Marilyn E. Parker*	15-2548	29.95	26.95
☐ **Annual Review of Women's Health, Volume II** *Edited by Beverly McElmurry* *& Randy Spreen Parker*	19-2669	37.95	34.35
☐ **Nursing Centers: The Time Is Now** *Edited by Barbara Murphy*	41-2629	25.95	22.95